Breast Cancer:

A Guide for Fellows

Breast Cancer:
A Guide for Fellows

Orlando E. Silva, M.D.

Medical Hematology and Oncology
236 Valencia Avenue
Coral Gables, FL 33134
USA

Stefano Zurrida, M.D.

Istituto Europeo di Oncologia
Direzione Scientifica
Via Ripamonti 435
20141 Milan
Italy

Presented by Umberto Veronesi, M.D.

1999

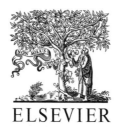

ELSEVIER

ELSEVIER
Amsterdam · Lausanne · New York · Oxford · Shannon · Singapore · Tokyo

ELSEVIER SCIENCE B.V.
Sara Burgerhartstraat 25
P.O. Box 211, 1000 AE Amsterdam, The Netherlands

First edition 1999

Reprinted from Critical Reviews in Oncology/Hematology, Vol. 29, No. 1/2.

Library of Congress Cataloging in Publication Data
A catalog record from the Library of Congress has beed applied for.

ISBN 0 444 50117 7

⊗ This paper used in this publication meets the requirements of ANSI/NISO Z39.48-1992 (Permanence of Paper).
Printed in The Netherlands.

Dedication

We dedicate this handbook to

The Fallen and The Standing Victims

along the way.

Here's to the Wives,

and the Mothers,

the Sisters and the Daughters

who made a difference

and guided the way.

Thank you.

We are still trying.

Orlando Silva

The authors would like to thank the following experts for actively participating and offering advice in the preparation of this handbook.

Umberto Veronesi, M.D.
Scientific Director
Istituto Europeo di Oncologia
Milan, Italy

Gabriel Hortobagyi, M.D.
Professor of Medicine
Chairman, Department of Breast Medical
  Oncology
MD Anderson Cancer Cener
Houston Texas, USA

James J. Vredenburgh, M.D.
Associate Professor of Medicine
Division of Medical Oncology
Duke University Medical Center
Durham, North Carolina, USA

Phillip Nicholas Blondeel, M.D., Ph.D.
Associate Professor Plastic Surgery
Department of Plastic Surgery and
  Reconstruction
University Hospital Gent
Gent, Belgium

Lawrence B. Marks, M.D.
Associate Professor of Radiation Oncology
Duke University Medical Center
Durham, North Carolina, USA

Giovanni Rosti, M.D.
Chairman, European Group for Blood and
  Marrow Transplantation
Solid Tumors Working Party
Division of Medical Oncology
Ospedale S. Maria delle Croci
Ravenna, Italy

Rex Bentley, M.D.
Assistant Professor of Pathology
Duke University Medical Center
Durham, North Carolina, USA

Robin T. Vollmer, M.D.
Assistant Professor of Pathology
Duke University Medical Center
Durham, North Carolina, USA

Eric P. Winer, M.D.
Director, Breast Oncology Center
Dana Farber Cancer Institute
Boston, Massachusetts, USA

Giammaria Fiorentini, M.D.
Secretary of International Society of   Regional
Cancer Treatment
Chief, Locoregional Cancer Therapy Unit
Division of Medical Oncology

Ospedale S. Maria delle Croci
Ravenna, Italy

William P. Peters, M.D.
President and CEO
Karmanos Cancer Center
Wayne State University
Detroit, Michigan, USA

Phyllis J. Kornguth, M.D.
Associate Professor of Radiology
Division of Breast Imaging
Duke University Medical Center
Durham, North Carolina, USA

George S. Leight, Jr., M.D.
Professor of Surgery
Division of General and Thoracic Surgery
Duke University Medical Center
Durham, North Carolina, USA

Annie Lindsay Drapkin, M.D.
Department of Obstetrics and Gynecology
Duke University Medical Center
Durham, North Carolina, USA

Maurizio Marangolo, M.D.
Chief of Medical Oncology Unit
Division of Medical Oncology
Ospedale S. Maria delle Croci
Ravenna, Italy

Barbara L. Fowble, M.D.
Clinical Director
Department of Radiation Oncology
Assoc Dir. Breast Evaluation Center
Senior Member Fox Chase Cancer Center
Philadelphia, Pennsylvania, USA

Eva Rubin, M.D.
Professor of Radiology
Mammography Section
University of Alabama
Birmingham, Alabama, USA

Carolyn Sartor, M.D.
Assistant Professor Radiation Oncology
Lineberger Cancer Center
University of North Carolina Medical
  School
Chapel Hill, North Carolina, USA

Special thanks to Nancy Winter who skillfully
typed this book, verified all the reference citations
and cheerfully endured and word-processed the
many updates and edits.

Foreword

I first became interested in breast cancer 40 years ago. During this long period I have seen the terrible progression of this disease that occurs in many patients, but also the tremendous progress that had been made in treating it. I am privileged to be part of the army that has won major battles against breast cancer. With increased public awareness of the disease, early detection procedures, the use of radiation, chemical and hormone therapies, as well as new surgical techniques, we have been able to improve overall survival and disease-free survival for women with this disease. We have also improved the quality of life by lowering local recurrence rates and by using less drastic surgical techniques such as quadrantectomy combined with radiation, instead of mutilating mastectomy. Much of this progress has been made by challenging established medical ideas with new evidence and new studies; along the way some views have been confirmed and others have been discarded.

This gem of a book, aimed at primary care physicians, oncology fellows and practicing oncologists, provides a digest of our current knowledge on breast cancer in a well-organized and easily accessible form. It is not an encyclopedic review but a handbook providing summaries of current thinking (not skirting areas of controversy), explanations, comprehensive references and above all, treatment options. The book references the most important articles in all areas of breast cancer; including not only the landmark studies in each section but also comprehensive and up-to-date review articles. It is the authors' intention that the book be useful 'close to the bedside'. I believe they have fulfilled their intention magnificently.

Umberto Veronesi
Scientific Director,
European Institute of Oncology, Milano

How to use this book

This handbook is written to be a useful 'bedside' reference to physicians in all specialties as well as a compendium of breast cancer information for nurses, medical students, clinical researchers and educators.

A special feature of this book is the table of contents which has been prepared as a literature outline, embedding in it all the citations. By this method the reader is provided with the references for the most current studies and trials, landmark articles, and review publications on many of the topics and subtopics relating to breast cancer.

The handbook is written in outline format to highlight the key concepts. Landmark and current clinical trials have been summarised into 5–10 lines, addressing whether the study was randomized, the number of women entered, over what period of time, the median follow-up, the results and the conclusions.

In addition, there is a comprehensive alphabetical index so the information required can be found quickly for your patient at the bedside. The various names for conditions are cross-referenced and the generic and brand names for the chemotherapeutic agents are supplied.

It is our hope that this publication will not only help the physician in patient care, but also help the physician scientist see where we are and where we might target research objectives in the near future. Our plan is to continue in this format and to publish periodic updates on the progress of the clinical research in this important area of medicine.

COMMONLY USED ABBREVIATIONS

ABMT	Autologous bone marrow transplant
b.i.d.	Twice a day
BMT	Bone marrow transplant
c.i.	Continuous infusion
CNS	Central nervous system
CR	Complete response
CSF	Cerebral spinal fluid
CT	Computerized tomography
DCIS	Ductal carcinoma in situ
DFS	Disease free survival
DVT	Deep venous thrombosis
EIC	Extensive intraductal component
ER	Estrogen receptor
FDA	Food and drug administration (USA)
HR	Hormone receptor
i.m.	Intramuscular
i.t.	Intrathecal
I.U.	International units
i.v.	Intravenous
LCIS	Lobular carcinoma in situ
LFT's	Liver function tests
LN	Lymph nodes
ml	Milliliter
MRM	Modified radical mastectomy
NCI	National cancer institute
OS	Overall survival
p.o.	By mouth
PE	Physical examination
PR	Progesterone receptor
q	Every
q.d.	Every day
rbc/hpf	Red blood cells per high powered field
r/o	Rule out
R.O.S.	Review of systems
s/p	Status post
TAM	Tamoxifen
t.i.d.	Three times a day
U.S.	United States of America
vs	Versus, or compared to
WBC	White blood cell count
XRT	Radiation therapy
♀	Woman or female

Table of contents

[Harris JR (ed) Diseases of the Breast. 1996].

- Benign breast tissue is heterogenous, containing fat, stroma, ducts and lobules.

Cysts

- Definition:
  — Fluid filled structures.
  — Derived from terminal duct lobular unit.

- Types:
  — Flattened.
  — Apocrine–(recurrence more likely).

- Location:
  — Cysts tend to be peripheral, occurring within the terminal duct or lobule.
  — Carcinoma generally occurs deeper in the breasts.

- Treatment:
  — Aspiration.
    — Management for symptomatic cysts.
    — Diagnosis in asymptomatic cysts.

- Cytology of aspirated fluid, if clear, is not necessary due to low yield in diagnosing cancer.

- [Bruzzi P. Br Med J 314: 925–928, 1997].
  — ♀ with gross cystic disease underwent breast cyst aspiration.
  — Cysts were classified according to cationic content.
    — Type I (K:Na > 1.5).
    — Type II (K:Na < 1.5).
    — Mixed.
  — Median follow-up: 6 years.
  — Incidence of breast cancer was significantly higher in ♀ with Type I cysts.
  — The relationship between the electrolyte content within the cyst and the risk of developing cancer needs further study.

Fibrocystic changes

● Are not a distinct entity.

● Heterogenous group of abnormalities often found together.
 — Cystic change.
 — Apocrine metaplasia.
 — Fibrosis.
 — Chronic inflammation.

● Clinical presentation:
 — Painless or painful palpable breast mass that fluctuates with menstrual cycles.
 — If proliferation is absent there is no association with breast carcinoma.

● Breast pain.
 — Avoid caffeine and chocolate.
 — Primrose oil.
  — In Wales they have found success with this treatment.
  — May also help with vasomotor symptoms.
  — It contains linoleic acid which functions as an anti-inflammatory agent, stabilizing adenyl cyclase in the breast.
  — Dose: 2000–3000 mg per day.
  — Randomized clinical trials are needed.

Epithelial hyperplasia
[Dupont WD, New Engl J Med 312: 146–151, 1985].

● Mild, moderate or florid proliferation of ductal cells.

● If moderate or florid, the relative risk of subsequently developing breast cancer is increased to 1.6 ×, and if there is a (+) family history, to 2 ×.

Atypical hyperplasia

● Proliferative lesions of the breast.

● Increases the relative risk of subsequently developing breast cancer ~ 4 × that of the general population and to 8.9 × with a (+) family history.
[Dupont WD, New Engl J Med 312: 146–151, 1985].

- Atypical ductal hyperplasia.
  - Shares features with DCIS.
  - In NSABP-B17, 7% of the cases diagnosed as DCIS were found on central review to be atypical ductal hyperplasia.

- Atypical lobular hyperplasia.
  - Shares features with LCIS.

Adenomas

- Well circumscribed tumors.

- Morphology may overlap with that of fibroadenoma.

- Types:
  - Tubular adenomas.
    - Affect young ♀.
    - Freely moveable nodules.
    - Clinically resemble fibroadenoma.

  - Lactating adenomas.
    - One or more freely moveable masses during pregnancy or post-partum, show marked secretory activity histologically.

  - Adenomas of the nipple.
    - Also known as 'florid papillomatosis' of the nipple ducts.
    - Usually present in ♀ 40–50 years of age, with nipple pain and bloody discharge.
    - Have been reported in association with carcinoma.
    - Careful search for ipsilateral cancer is warranted.
    - Treatment:
      - Excision.

Fibroadenoma
[Dupont WD, New Engl J Med, 331: 10–15, 1994].

- Common cause of benign breast mass in young ♀.
  - Most common cause of benign breast mass in adolescence.

- ~ 10% are bilateral.

- Pathology:
  - No true capsule.
  - Proliferation of both the stroma and the ducts.
  - May express estrogen/progesterone receptors.

- Common finding on mammogram.
  - 'Popcorn' calcifications.

- May become very large-giant fibroadenoma.
  - Infarction can occur most commonly during pregnancy and lactation, causing a discrete breast mass.

- Treatment:
  - Excise completely with wide margins to avoid recurrence.
  - If older than 35 years old, remove because of risk of phyllodes.
  - If 25–35 years old, need good cytology → fine needle aspiration (FNA).
    - Core biopsy can be an alternative.
    - Follow without surgery, unless it is causing the patient problems.
  - Infrequently, fibroadenoma may occur in association with carcinoma, most commonly LCIS (65%).

Mammary duct ectasia

- Also known as periductal mastitis.

- Occurs when intraductal content extravasates into periductal tissue.

- Definition:
  - Dilated subareolar ducts, usually ruptured, associated with chronic inflammation and fibrosis.

- Clinical manifestations:
  - Subareolar tenderness.
  - Hard mass.
  - Nipple discharge from several ducts (may be bloody).
  - Nipple inversion (may be also observed in breast carcinoma).
  - Chronic fistulas may develop.
  - When acute, mimics breast abcess.

- Occurs primarily in perimenopausal and postmenopausal ♀.
  - Most commonly occurs in fourth decade of life.
  - Not a disease; a condition.
  - May or may not be radiographically evident.
  - Very common finding with mammography.
    - Spherical and tubular calcifications in dilated ducts.
    - Calcifications are often large, uniform and bilateral.
    - The borders of the individual calcifications are smooth.

- Smoking and bacteria (especially anaerobic) play a role in its etiology. [Dixon JM, Br J Surg 83: 820–822, 1996].

- Neither parity nor breast feeding play a role in its etiology. [Dixon JM, Br J Surg 70: 60–63, 1983].

- Treatment:
  - Patients with mass → biopsy to rule out malignancy.
  - Needle biopsy is often sterile.
  - Patients with discharge → excise dilated subareolar duct to rule out malignancy.
  - Broad spectrum antibiotics to cover anaerobes.
    - Amoxicillin-clavulanic acid (Augmentin).
    - For penicillin-allergic patients, erythromycin and metronidazole.

Mammary duct fistula

- Most commonly develops as a complication of duct ectasia.

- Treatment:
  - Excise fistula and duct up to nipple.
  - Provide broad spectrum antibiotics.
  - Pathogen: anaerobes.

Papillomas

- Definition:
  - Proliferation of epithelium or arborescent stalks supported by a fibrocapsular core. If it lacks a core, then it is micropapillary.
  - Tumors of lactiferous ducts or terminal ductal-lobular unit.

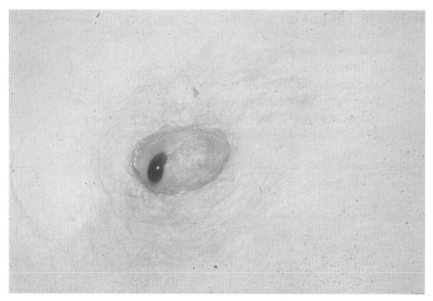

Fig. 1. Frankly bloody discharge from nipple, suggesting the presence of intraductal papilloma.

● Types:
  — Solitary intraductal papilloma
    — Most commonly ♀ 30–50 years of age.
    — Most commonly presents with bloody nipple discharge (Fig. 1), may also present as a palpable mass close to the areola.
    — Usually occur centrally in the large subareolar ducts.
    — Generally < 1 cm in size.
      — May encyst, producing masses as large as 10 cm.
    — May be difficult to distinguish from papillary carcinoma histologically.
    — May undergo infarction.
    — Treatment:
      — Total duct excision.
      — Slightly increased risk of subsequent breast cancer.

  — Multiple papillomas.
    — Also known as papillomatosis and multiple peripheral papillomas.
    — <u>NOT</u> to be confused for epithelial hyperplasia.
    — Usually occur in younger ♀.

— Typically presents as a breast mass.
— Less often presents with nipple discharge.
— Often bilateral.
— Most frequently peripheral in location arising within the terminal duct lobular unit.
— High local recurrence rate.
— Susceptible to malignant transformation.
  — This is related to the presence of associated hyperplasia.
  — If <u>no</u> hyperplasia, <u>no</u> risk of cancer.
— Treatment:
  — Complete excision with diligent follow-up of both breasts.

Puerperal (lactational) mastitis

• Acute cellulitis of the lactating breast.

• Clinical manifestations:
— Warm, red, tender breast.
— Fevers, chills.

• If untreated, may progress to an abscess.
— Commonly occurs during early weeks of nursing.
— Increased WBC/ml in milk.

• Types:

— Sporadic form.
  — Infant does not harbor pathogen.
  — Most common pathogen.
    — *Staphylococcus aureus.*

— Treatment:
  — Antibiotics (penicillin, dicloxacillin, erythromycin).
  — Encourage patient to continue breast feeding to prevent milk stasis and breast engorgement.
  — Apply manual pressure and warmth to the area.
  — Infant not affected by nursing from affected breast.

— Epidemic form.
  — Infant harbors the pathogen orally.
  — Also known as acute mammary adenitis.
  — Uncommon.
  — Occurs in hospitals/maternity wards.
  — Most common pathogen: *S. aureus.*

— Treatment:
  — Antibiotics, as above.
  — Manual pressure and warmth.
  — Pumping of affected breast.
  — Weaning is necessary since the infant harbors the pathogen.

Periareolar sepsis

- Nonpuerperal (non-lactational) breast abscess
  — Most common breast abscess.
  — Usually occurs in subareolar area.
  — Often indolent and relapsing.
  — Patient generally not systemically toxic.
  — Affects both males and females.

- Pathogen.
  — Think anaerobes (bacteroides, peptostreptococcus, propionibacterium).

- Treatment:
  — Incision and drainage with broad spectrum antibiotic coverage during the acute phase.
    — Antibiotics → metronidazole, augmentin (amoxicillin-clavulanic acid).
  — Biopsy the wall of the abscess cavity to rule out malignancy.
  — After resolution of acute event.
    — Excise the major duct system beneath the areola (Hadfield procedure).

- Puerperal (lactational) breast abscess
  — May result from untreated puerperal mastitis.
  — If tenderness and erythema of the puerperal mastitis do not resolve promptly after appropriate antibiotic coverage, must rule out abscess.

— Treatment:
  — Incision and drainage over point of maximal tenderness with biopsy of the abscess wall to rule out malignancy.
  — Broad spectrum antibiotics.
  — Healing is prompt, fistula formation is rare.

Fat necrosis

● May simulate carcinoma clinically and/or mammographically.

● Clinical manifestation:
  — Painless, firm, irregular mass often in a superficial part of the breast; skin retraction may occur.

● Most commonly occurs in heavy-set, middle-aged ♀ with large pendulous breasts.

● Associated with trauma, surgery, and radiation therapy to the breast.

● Diagnosis:
  — By FNA or biopsy.

Mondor disease

● Phlebitis of the thoracoepigastric vein.

● May occur after trauma, surgery, or radiation to the breast.

● Clinical manifestations (Fig. 2):
  — Visible cord-like vein.
  — May cause skin retraction.
  — Pain along the course of the thoracoepigastric vein that runs from the axilla laterally across the breast to the subareolar area where it crosses medially and then extends to the epigastrium.

● Benign and limited.

Granular cell tumors

● Simulate carcinoma on presentation and on mammogram.

● More common among African Americans.

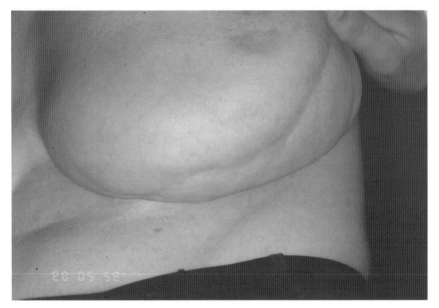

Fig. 2. Mondor disease: sometimes this is the first sign of breast cancer.

- Typically presents between puberty and menopause.

- Typically located in the upper inner quadrant as opposed to carcinoma which occurs most commonly in the upper outer quadrant.

- The granules are secondary lysosomes seen on electron microscopy.

- Generally benign.

- Treatment:
  — Wide excision—can recur locally.

Lipomas

- Consist of encapsulated nodules of adipose tissue.

Hamartomas (Fibroadenolipoma)

- Uncommon breast lesions.

- Clinical manifestations:
  — Palpable breast mass.
  — Often poorly palpable.

- May be an incidental finding during surgery.

- Closely resemble normal breast histology.
  — Encapsulated area of normal breast tissue.

Sarcoid

- Breast involvement is rare.

- Clinically may simulate carcinoma.

- Pathology:
  — Non-caseating granulomata.

BREAST CARCINOMA

HISTORY OF BREAST CANCER

2000 BC–1840 AD

- 1600 BC: First description of breast cancer appears in an ancient Egyptian papyrus housed in the British Museum.

- 400 BC: Hippocrates; Greece, describes case report of breast cancer.

- 200 AD: Galen; Rome, described blood vessels, resembling crab's legs surrounding a breast tumor.
  - He thought breast cancer was due to a coagulum of black bile within the breast.
  - Therapy was aimed at getting rid of the excess black bile by diets, purgation, venesection, cupping and leeching.
  - Unchallenged until the early 19th century.

1810–1987

- 1810: Muller described the cellular nature of cancer.

- 1840: Virchow hypothesized the tumor arose in the epithelial cells of the breast and invaded locally and centrifugally in all directions.

- 1889: Halsted performed the first radical mastectomy.
  - Believed breast cancer was an orderly disease spreading in a contiguous fashion from the primary site via the lymphatics.

- 1894: Halsted reported the results of the first radical mastectomy series at Johns Hopkins.

- 1896: Sir George Thomas Beatson demonstrated how surgical removal of ovaries can lead to therapeutic response in metastatic breast cancer.

- 1906: Louis Ombredanne was the first to describe the pectoral muscle flap for immediate mound reconstruction.

- 1930s: Sir Jeffrey Keynes of St. Bartholomew's Hospital
  - Systemic hypothesis: breast cancer is a systemic disease and lymph node involvement is not orderly.

— Introduced tumourectomy and radium needle insertions.
— The 5-year survival rates were very similar to those achieved by radical mastectomy.

- 1940s: Sir Stanford Cade concluded that in stage I disease the best method of treatment was radical mastectomy.

- 1948: Dr Patey develops modified radical mastectomy.

- Throughout the first 65 years of this century, radical mastectomy was the treatment of choice.

- 1960: Dr Bernard Fisher and Dr Ed Fisher of Pittsburgh, Dr Devitt of Ottawa, and Dr Crile of the Cleveland Clinic provided experimental evidence which contradicted the teachings of Dr Halsted and Dr Virchow.
  — Cancer cells usually did not spread in a predictable centrifugal manner along lymphatics.

- 1987: Dr Samuel Hellman and Dr J. Harris proposed the spectrum hypothesis.
  — Breast cancer presents as a spectrum of disease from local disease to systemic disease when first detected.
  — Stresses the importance of both local and systemic therapy.

EPIDEMIOLOGY
[Hortobagyi GN, CA Cancer J Clin 45: 199–226, 1995].
[Harris JR, New Engl J Med 327(5): 319–328, 1992].

- Incidence is four to five times higher in North America and Northern Europe than in Asia and Africa.

- The incidence in the USA has been increasing steadily since 1960 at a rate of 1–2% per year.

- Breast cancer is the most common cancer in American ♀, accounting for 32% of all cancer in ♀.

- The overall incidence of breast cancer in Japan is ~ 1/5th that of the USA.
  - Incidence among Asian and Japanese immigrants to the USA remains unchanged; however, among their descendants, it has increased to USA rates.

- In the UK there are ~ 26 000 new cases per year.

- In USA ~ 183 000 new cases per year.
  - The American Cancer Society estimates ~ 180 000 new cases for 1997.

- In the USA, ~ 44 000 deaths occurred in 1995, ~ 44 300 deaths occurred in 1996, and ~ 43 900 deaths occurred in 1997.

- 1/15 ♀ (7%) in Western Europe will develop breast cancer during their lifetime.

- 1/8 ♀ (12%) in USA will develop breast cancer during their lifetime.
  - 12% of USA ♀, will develop it if they live to be 85 years old.
  - 50% of the patient's risk occurs after age 65.
  - 6.5% of all breast cancer occurs in ♀ < 40 years of age.
  - So there is no current breast cancer crisis attacking young ♀.

- Breast cancer is the leading cause of death among USA women 40–55 years of age.

- Breast cancer is the 2nd highest cancer killer of American women (2nd only to lung cancer in the USA).

- Increases have occurred in all age groups since 1935, although the magnitude of the increase has been greatest among older women.

- 21% rise in incidence occurred between 1973 and 1990.
  - Cannot be explained entirely by mammographic screening.

- Mortality rates have decreased in the USA.
  - 2000–3000 fewer deaths per year.
  - This has also been documented in Europe (Sweden).

— This decline seems to be related mainly to a decrease in the mortality of young ♀.
— Is it due to earlier detection?
  — Mammogram on general population decreases mortality rates by ∼ 20%.
  — Adjuvant therapy on general population decreases mortality rates by ∼ 20%.
  — Probably the combination of these two factors have played a key role.

- Age at diagnosis.
  [Nixon AJ, J Clin Oncol 12: 888–894, 1994].
  [Albain KS, J Natl Cancer Inst Monogr 16: 35–42, 1994].
  — Two large studies have found patients younger than 35 years of age have a worse prognosis than older patients.
  — There are studies, however, that have found no relation with age.

- Ethnicity.
  [Elledge RM, J Natl Cancer Inst 86: 705–712, 1994].
  — Breast cancer survival rate is poorer among black and hispanic ♀ than among white ♀.
  [Moormeier J, Ann Int Med 124(10): 897–905, 1996].
  — The incidence of postmenopausal breast cancer is lower in black and hispanic ♀ than it is in white ♀.
    — Breast cancer at a young age is more common in black ♀ than white ♀.
  — Breast tumors in black ♀ are diagnosed at a more advanced stage of disease.
  — Black ♀ have a higher frequency of poorly differentiated tumors and a lower frequency of hormone receptor (+) tumors.
  — 5 year survival rate for black ♀ is 64% vs. that of white ♀ that is 80%.

- Laterality.
  [Weiss HA, Cancer Causes Control 7: 539–543, 1996].
  — In the USA breast cancer is more likely to occur in the left breast.

- Most ♀ (∼ 66%) that develop breast cancer do not have major risk factors.

- ♀ with breast cancer have an increased risk of developing another breast cancer, as well as ovarian and colon cancer.

RISK FACTORS
[Harris JR, New Engl J Med 327(5): 319–328, 1992].

- ~ 66% ♀ with breast cancer have no known risk factors.

Factors that increase risk
[Bilimoria MM, CA Cancer J Clin: 45: 263–278, 1995].

- Gender.
  - # 1 risk factor.
  - ♀:♂ = 100:1.

- Age.
  - ♀, 35 years → 65 years old: as age progresses, there is 6-fold increase in breast cancer.
  - At age 60, ~ 17 of every 1000 ♀ are expected to develop breast cancer within 5 years.

- Hormonal factors.
  [Brinton LA, Cancer Invest 6: 245–254, 1988].
  - General rule:
    - Uninterrupted menstrual cycling for long periods of time ↑ risk.

  - Menstrual history:
    - Early menarche.
      - In China the average age of menarche is 17 years.
      - In the USA the average age of menarche is 12.8 years.
    - Regular menses.
      [Henderson BE, Cancer 56: 1206–1208, 1985].
      - Establishing regular menstrual cycles within 1 year of the first menstrual period.
    - Late menopause.
      [Trichopoulos D, J Natl Cancer Inst 48: 605–613, 1972].
      - ♀ who experienced menopause before age 45 are estimated to have one-half the breast cancer risk of ♀ who experienced menopause after age 55.
    - Irregularity of menstrual cycles.
      - May be protective [Parazzini F, Oncology 50: 222–225, 1993].

- Reproductive history:
  - Nulliparity ↓ risk by 30%.
  - ♀ whose first full term pregnancy > 25 year old have 40% ↑ risk vs. ♀ that have first full term pregnancy at age ≤ 20.
    [Lambe M, New Engl J Med 331: 5–9, 1994].
    - There appears to be a transient ↑ risk of breast cancer after giving birth.
    - This risk is more pronounced for ♀ who have their first child at a later age.
- Diethylstilbestrol (DES) use in pregnancy.

- In premenopausal ♀, long term exogenous estrogen use is controversial.
  - Two meta-analyses have failed to demonstrate a substantially ↑ risk.
    [Schlesselman JJ, Contraception 40: 1–38, 1989].
    - There appears to be a small but real risk for young ♀ using birth control pills, especially before their first pregnancy.

- In postmenopausal ♀, hormone replacement is controversial.
  [Colditz GA, New Engl J Med 332: 1589–1593, 1995].
  - Prospective cohort study.
  - In ♀ taking hormone replacement for more than 5 years (estrogen alone or estrogen + progestin) the risk of breast cancer was significantly increased over ♀ not taking any hormonal replacement.
  - The risk was also greatest in ♀ older than 60 years old receiving hormonal therapy.
  - The addition of progestins to estrogen does not reduce the risk of breast cancer in this population.
  - This study confirmed previous European studies.
    [Bergkvist L, New Engl J Med 321: 293–297, 1989].
  - Conclusion: hormone replacement should be recommended only on an individual patient basis weighing risk-benefit issues of breast cancer vs. that of heart disease and osteoporosis.

- Oral contraceptives.
  [Collaborative Group on Hormonal Factors in Breast Cancer: Lancet 347: 1713–1727, 1996].
  - Pooled analysis from 54 epidemiologic studies.
  - Current users of oral contraceptives had a small, but independent, ↑ risk when compared to ♀ who had never used them.

- The risk of breast cancer ↓ steadily after discontinuing the use of oral contraceptives.
  - After 10 years of discontinuation, the risk of past users became equal to the risk of ↓ who had never used them.

- Atypical epithelial hyperplasia.
  [Dupont WD, Cancer 71: 1258–1265, 1993].
  - ↑ risk especially if positive family history
    [Dupont WD, New Engl J Med 312: 146–151, 1985].
  - If present in a patient with breast cancer in a 1st degree relative: ↑ risk 8–12 × .
  - ♀ with atypical hyperplasia have a 4 × ↑ risk of developing breast cancer.
  - ♀ with moderate to florid hyperplasia without atypia, have a 2 × ↑ risk of developing breast cancer.
  - The cancer risk is bilateral and equally likely to occur in either breast.
  - It is uncertain if the risk remains constant over time.
    - It may ↓ after ∼ 10 years.
  - There is no relationship between fibrocystic changes of the breast without proliferation and breast cancer.

- Previous history of cancer.
  - ♀ with a personal history of endometrial or ovarian carcinoma have 2 × ↑ risk of breast cancer over that of normal ♀.
  - Breast carcinomas in situ: DCIS/LCIS.
  - An association has been reported among ♀ with melanoma or salivary gland tumors and breast carcinoma.

- Previous breast cancer.
  - 5-Fold ↑.
  - Continued screening of these patients is imperative.
  - These ♀ also have an ↑ risk of developing endometrial, ovarian, and colon carcinomas.

- The lifetime risk of a contralateral primary breast cancer is increased by:
  - Youth at diagnosis of the first lesion.
  - Family history of bilateral breast cancer.
  - Presence of lobular carcinoma in situ.

- Ionizing radiation.
  [Bhatia S, New Engl J Med 334: 745–751, 1996].
  [John EM, Epidemiol Rev 15: 157–62, 1993].
  - Especially dangerous between puberty and age 30.
    - Peak incidence if exposure took place between 15–18 years of age.
    - No ↑ risk if exposure occurs after age 40, so mammograms do not ↑ risk.
  - Atomic bomb exposure (100 rad) → 3 × ↑ risk of breast cancer.
  - ♀ with a previous history of Hodgkin's disease treated with irradiation.
    - Breast cancer in Hodgkin's patients tends to occur at younger age, medial segments, and more often bilateral.
      [Yahalom J, J Clin Oncol 10: 1674–1681, 1992].
    - Patients must undergo screening mammogram beginning at age 35 or 10 years after therapy, whichever comes first.

- Alcohol.
  [Smith-Warner SA, J Am Med Assoc 279: 535–540, 1998].
  [Longnecker MP, Cancer Causes Control 5: 73–82, 1994].
  [Longnecker MP, J Am Med Assoc 260: 652–656, 1988].
  [Willett WC, New Engl J Med 316: 1174–1180, 1987].
  [Tannenbaum A, Cancer Research 2: 468–475, 1942].
  - Two drinks/day, ↑ risk (1.4–1.7 ×).
  - The source of alcohol does seem to influence the breast cancer risk.

- Family history.
  - 85% do not have family history of breast cancer.
  - If mother, sister, or daughter have (+) history of breast cancer, the patient's risk is increased 2-fold (sister > mother).
  - If two 1st degree relatives have breast cancer, the patient's risk is 25 ± 11% or 4–6-fold increase and even as high as 50% if one of the two relatives have bilateral disease before 50 years of age.

- Hereditary breast cancer.
  [Greene MH, Mayo Clin Proc 72: 54–65, 1997].
  [Contemporary Oncology Jan 1994, 4: 23–31].
  - ∼ 5–10% of all breast cancers have an inherited basis.
  - All are autosomal dominant and most are bilateral.
  - Males carry the deleterious gene 50% of the time.
  - Carriers of germline mutation have a 4% per year risk of developing breast cancer. [Verhoog LC, Lancet 351: 316–321, 1998].

— BRCA1 and BRCA2 are tumor-suppressor genes that when mutated are associated with a much higher risk of developing breast and ovarian cancer.
   — BRCA1 and BRCA2 encode for proteins whose fundamental role is DNA repair.
   — ♀ who inherit a single mutated copy of either BRCA1 or BRCA2 have a significantly ↑ lifetime risk of breast cancer.
   [Ford D, Lancet 343: 692–695, 1994].

— ∼ 45 years of age is the median to develop inherited breast cancer (BRCA1/BRCA2).
— When obtaining the patient's family history, it is important elicit:
   — The age of onset of breast cancer in the afflicted family member (it is more important than the actual number of ♀ in the family who have developed breast cancer);
   — If there has been a history of breast cancer on the father's side of the family, and if there has been any ovarian cancer in the family.

— <u>BRCA1</u>
   — Accounts for ∼ 30–40% of all inherited breast cancer.
   — A gene for early-onset breast cancer and breast-ovarian cancer.
   — Autosomal dominant with high penetrance.
   — BRCA1 transcription factor recently discovered.
   — Mapped to a region on chromosome 17 (17q21).
   — 85% lifetime risk of developing breast cancer.
   — Associated risk: 50% by age 50
                          87% by age 70 (85% lifetime risk).
                  vs.
   General population risk: 2% by age 50
                          7% by age 70.
   — ↑ risk of developing a 2nd breast primary by age 70 if survives the first.
   — 40–50% risk of developing ovarian cancer.
      — But it does not occur at an earlier age.
   — [Rubin SC, New Engl J Med 335: 1413–1416, 1996].
      — Ovarian cancer in BRCA1 mutation may have a more favorable clinical course than sporadic ovarian cancer in the general population.
   — Breast cancer gene inheritance can be maternal or paternal.
   — Male carriers do not develop breast cancer, although they are at ↑ risk of developing colon cancer (4 × ↑) and prostate cancer (3 × ↑).

[Langston AA, New Engl J Med 334: 137–142, 1996].
— 80 ♀, in whom breast cancer was diagnosed before age 35 and
  who were not selected on the basis of family history, were
  studied.
— BRCA1 alterations were identified in ~ 10% of the ♀.

[FitzGerald MG, New Engl J Med 334: 143–149, 1996].
— Peripheral blood samples were obtained on 418 ♀ diagnosed
  with breast cancer before the age of 40, in the Boston area.
    — Germ line BRCA1 mutations can be present in young ♀ with
      breast cancer who do not have a family history of cancer.
    — The specific BRCA1 mutation, 185delAG, is strongly
      associated with the onset of breast cancer before the age of
      40, among Jewish ♀ of central European (Ashkenazi) origin,
      with a frequency of ~ 1–2%, as opposed to ~ 0.1% in
      unselected Caucasian population.
    [Struewing JP, New Engl J Med 336: 1401–1408, 1997].

— BRCA2
[Krainer M, New Engl J Med 336: 1416–1421, 1997].
[Nature Genetics 8: 105–106, 1994].
— A second breast cancer gene has been mapped to chromosome
  13 (13q12-13).
— Early onset breast cancer in ♀.
— 85% lifetime risk.
— No ↑ risk of ovarian cancer for carriers.
— ↑ Risk of cancer of the uterus (4 ×).
— ↑ Risk male breast cancer (15 ×).
— ↑ Risk of prostate cancer (4 ×) and at an earlier age.
[Neuhausen S, Nat Genet 13: 126–128, 1996].
— The specific BRCA2 mutation, 6174delT, is present in Ashkenazi
  Jews, but the frequency of breast cancer related to this specific
  mutation is lower than BRCA1 and other BRCA2 mutations.
    — Occurs in ~ 1% of Ashkenazi Jews.
    — The BRCA1 185delAG mutation is 4 × more common
      among Ashkenazi ♀ with breast cancer than is the BRCA2
      6174delT mutation.
[Thorlacius S, Nat Genet 13: 117–119, 1996].
— The specific BRCA2 mutation, 999del15, occurs among
  Icelanders.

- A genetically isolated population, similar to the Ashkenazi Jews.
- An estimated 40% of all male breast cancer in Iceland is attributable to this mutation.

- Familial breast and colon cancer
  - Transmission is autosomal dominant with high penetrance.

- Li-Fraumeni syndrome
  [Li FP, Ann Intern Med 71: 747–752, 1969].
  [Strong LC, Am J Epidemiol 135: 190–199, 1992].
  - Transmission is autosomal dominant with high penetrance.
  - Associated with abnormal p53 tumor-suppressor gene (germline mutation).
    - Inactivation of one allele is required for inhibition, unlike in the classic tumor suppressor gene (retinoblastoma gene) in which inactivation of both alleles is required.
    - Direct testing is possible for this condition.
  - Presents as early onset breast cancer.
  - Members of these families have a higher than expected incidence of breast cancer, sarcomas, brain tumors, lung cancer, leukemias, and adrenocortical cancers at early age.
  - RB-1
    - A tumor suppressor gene that is altered in ~ 15–20% of breast cancers.
    [Fung YK, Cancer Treat Res 61: 59–68, 1992].
    - The loss of RB gene is frequently accompanied by the loss of the p53 gene.

- Cowden's disease (multiple hamartoma syndrome)
  [Lloyd KM, Ann Intern Med 58: 136–142, 1963].
  [Starink PM, Clin Genet 29: 222–233, 1986].
  - Transmission is autosomal dominant with variable penetrance.
  - Premenopausal breast cancer.
  - ~ 30% of affected ♀ have breast cancer, often bilateral and typically at a younger than average age.
  - The Cowden gene has been mapped to 10q22-23, although the gene itself has not yet been cloned. [Nelen MR, Nat Genet 13: 114–116, 1996].
  - < 200 cases in the literature.

- Syndrome:
  - Multiple hamartomas of skin and oral cavity.
  - Papillomatosis of the skin and oral mucosa.
  - Thyroid tumors.
    - Thyroid goiter.
    - Thyroid adenomas.
  - Vitiligo.
  - Gastrointestinal polyps.
  - Uterine leiomyomas and lipomas.
  - Benign breast lesions have also been noted.

- Muir syndrome
  [Muir EG, Br J Surg 54: 191–195, 1967].

  - Transmission is autosomal dominant with high penetrance.
  - Results from germline mutations in the MSH2 and MLH1 loci.
    - Genes involved in DNA repair.
  - Syndrome:
    - Basal cell carcinoma.
    - Benign and malignant GI tumors.
    - Breast cancer, mostly postmenopausal.

- Ataxia-telangiectasia (A.T.)
  [Swift M, New Engl J Med 325: 1831–1836, 1991].
  - Autosomal recessive.
  - Gene is mapped to chromosome 11q22-23. [Savitsky K, Science 268: 1749–1753, 1995].
  - Syndrome:
    - Progressive neurologic degeneration.
    - Cerebellar ataxia.
    - Oculocutaneous telangiectasias.
    - Radiation hypersensitivity.
    - Immunodeficiency.
    - Increased incidence of malignancy.
      - Especially non-Hodgkin's lymphoma.
  - Patients with A.T. are at an ↑ risk of developing breast cancer.
    - Heterozygote carriers have ↑ risk of breast cancer (5 ×).
  - ~ 1.4% of the population carry the gene (heterozygotes).

- Genetic testing.
  [Greene MH, Mayo Clin Proc 72: 54–65, 1998].
  [Statement of the American Society of Clinical Oncology, J Clin Oncol 14: 1730–1736, 1996].

  — Testing should be performed when:
    1. There is a high likelihood of a (+) test.
    2. The result can be adequately interpreted.
    3. The test results can influence medical management of the patient or family members.

  — Elements of the informed consent that should be reviewed with the patient:
    1. Confidentiality.
    2. Cost.
    3. Information on the specific test used and its technical accuracy.
    4. Implications of (+) or (−) test results.
    5. Risks of undergoing testing.

  — In the USA, The Health Insurance Portability and Accountability Act of 1996:
    — Prohibits group health plans from denying or limiting coverage based on genetic information; and
    — Provides protection against genetic discrimination.

- Current recommendations for high risk patients:
  — There are 3 options:
    1. Close surveillance.
       — Should begin 10 years younger than the youngest affected relative.
       — Monthly breast self examination, beginning in late teens.
       — Semi-annual clinical examinations starting at age 20.
       — Annual mammograms starting at age 25–35.
       — Semi-annual ovarian cancer screening with pelvic examination, transvaginal color doppler ultrasound and CA-125.

    2. Participation in chemo-prevention trials.

    3. Prophylactic bilateral complete mastectomies including the nipple-areola complex and the tail of Spence and prophylactic oophorectomies.

— At the completion of child-bearing or at the time of menopause.
— Subcutaneous mastectomies are inadequate procedures for prophylaxis.
— Prophylactic surgery minimizes, but does <u>NOT</u> completely eliminate the risk of developing breast or ovarian cancer, because it
  does not remove all normal tissue and because tumors may arise
  from peritoneum.

[Hartmann L, Proc Annu Meet Am Assoc Cancer Res 38: A1123, 1997].
— Chart review study.
— 2029 ♀ underwent bilateral or unilateral prophylactic mastectomies at
  the Mayo Clinic from 1960–1993.
— All the patient's next-of-kin were sent questionnaires to assess accurate risk factor and follow-up data.
— 1125 questionnaires have been completed to-date.
— They have been evaluated using a validated assessment tool (Gail
  Model).
— Preliminary findings suggest that prophylactic mastectomy significantly reduces the risk of breast cancer even in ♀ with a significant
  family history.

[Schrag D, New Engl J Med 336: 1465–1471, 1997]
— Prophylactic mastectomy is effective 85% of the time in patients with
  BRCA1.

— Conclusion:
  — Prophylactic mastectomy may ↓ but does <u>NOT</u> eliminate risk.
  — Prospective registry is needed.

Potential risk factors

● Diet.
  — Diet high in animal fat.
    — Data is weak at best
[Hunter DJ, New Engl J Med 334: 356–61, 1996].
— Analysis of the original data from 7 prospective studies, in standard-
  ized fashion.
— No evidence of a positive association between total dietary fat intake
  and the risk of breast cancer was found.

- Obesity.
  [Ursin G, Epidemiology 6: 137–141, 1995].
  [Kelsey JL, Epidemiol Rev 1: 74–109, 1979].
  [DeWaard F, Cancer 40: 1269–1275, 1977].
  – Obesity is a risk factor in postmenopausal ♀, however it seems protective in premenopausal ♀.
  [Huang Z, J Am Med Assoc 278: 1407–1411, 1997].
  – 95 256 US ♀ nurses studied, age 30–55 years old.
  – Followed for 16 years.
  – 2517 incidental breast cancers were documented.
    – 60% postmenopausal.
  – Higher body mass index at 18 years of age was associated with lower breast cancer incidence both before and after menopause.
  – Weight gain after 18 years of age was unrelated to breast cancer incidence before menopause, but was positively associated with the incidence of breast cancer after menopause.
    – The ↑ risk of breast cancer associated with weight gain was limited to ♀ who never used postmenopausal hormones.
    – Among these ♀, the relative risk was 1.99 (95% confidence interval), 1.43–2.76 for weight gain > 20 kg vs. unchanged weight.

- Organochlorine exposure (xenoestrogens).
  [Hunter DJ, New Engl J Med 337: 1253–1258, 1997].
  – Organochlorines are weakly estrogenic pollutants such as:
    – Polychlorinated biphenyls
    – DDT-pesticides.
    – DDE-pesticides.
  – 240 ♀ prospectively evaluated.
  – Organochlorine exposure in these ♀ did not ↑ risk of breast cancer.

Factors that decrease risk
[Lambe M, New Engl J Med 331: 5–9, 1994].

- Early age at first full term pregnancy.
  – Birth of first child before age 18.

- Physical activity.
  [Bernstein L, J Natl Cancer Inst. 86:1403–1408; 1994].
  – Cohort study with a median follow-up of 13 years.
  – Physical activity in adolescents and adults ↓ risk of breast cancer in ♀ up to 40 years of age.

[Thune I, New Engl J Med 336: 1269–1275, 1997].
- 25 624 Norwegian ♀ prospectively studied.
- All cases of breast cancer were identified over a median follow-up period of 13.7 years.
- A 37% ↓ risk of breast cancer (statistically significant) was found among ♀ who exercised regularly.
- The greatest benefit was seen in ♀ < 45 years old, who continued to exercise regularly over a period of 3–5 years.

[Rockhill B, J Natl Cancer Inst 90(15): 1155–1160, 1998].
- The Nurses Health Study did not find the same correlation between physical activity and breast cancer risk among young adult ♀.

- How to and how much exercise remains a question.

● Artificial menopause before age 35.
- Early oophorectomy.

● Lactation.
[Romieu I, Am J Epidemiol 143: 543–552, 1996].
[Newcomb PA, New Engl J Med 330: 81–87, 1994].
[Ross RK, New Engl J Med 330: 1683, 1994].
- After adjustment for parity, age at first delivery, and other risk factors for breast cancer, lactation was associated with a slight reduction in the risk of breast cancer among premenopausal women.
- Increasing cumulative duration of lactation was associated with a decreased risk of breast cancer among premenopausal women.
- A younger age at 1st lactation was significantly associated with a reduction in the risk of premenopausal breast cancer.
- No reduction in the risk of breast cancer occurred among postmenopausal women with a history of lactation.
- [Weiss HA, Epidemiology 8: 181–187, 1997].
  - Having been breast fed may protect against breast cancer.

● Abortion, spontaneous or induced, has no protective effect.

[Newcomb BE, J Am Med Assoc 275: 283–287, 1996].
- Population-based case-control study.
- 6888 ♀ younger than 75 years of age, recently diagnosed with breast cancer, were studied.

- A weak positive association was observed between abortion whether induced or spontaneous and the risk of breast cancer.
- Conclusion: to date the data is unclear.

[Melbye M, New Engl J Med 336: 81–85, 1997].
- Large cohort study.
- 1338 breast cancers diagnosed in ♀ who had terminated pregnancies.
- No association with early abortion (~ 7 weeks gestation) and breast cancer was found.

● Vitamin intake.
  - Questionable.

[Hunter DJ, New Engl J Med 329: 234–240, 1993].
- Vitamin A has been shown in some studies to reduce risk of breast cancer.
  - Not proven in large Randomized trials.
- Other antioxidants, such as vitamin C and vitamin E, have not been shown to be protective.

● Diet.
  - Questionable.

[Hunter DJ, New Engl J Med 334: 356–361, 1996].
[Willett WC, J Am Med Assoc 268: 2037–2044, 1992].
- Diets high in fiber have not been shown to be protective.

[Kaizer L, Nutr Cancer 12: 61–68, 1989].
- Diet rich in fish oils seem to be protective.
- Large Randomized studies are needed.

[Ingram D, Lancet 350(9083): 990–994, 1997].
- Phyto-estrogens.
  - Naturally occurring chemicals derived from plants.
  - Structure similar to estrogen.
  - Form part of our diet.
- Case-controlled study to evaluate the association between phyto-estrogen intake (measured by urinary excretion) and the risk of breast cancer.
- Age-matched controls were selected.

- 144 pairs were included for analysis.
- ♀ with newly diagnosed breast cancer, before receiving any treatment, gave a 72-h urine collection and a blood sample.
- After adjustment for age and menarche, parity, alcohol intake, and total fat intake, high excretion of phyto-estrogens, particularly the isoflavonic phyto-estrogen equol and the lignan enterolactone, was associated with a substantial ↓ in breast cancer risk.
- These findings could be important in the prevention of breast cancer.

[Lee HP, Lancet 337: 1197–1200, 1991].
- Diets rich in soybean products seem to be protective.
- Large Randomized trials are needed.

SCREENING

[Harris J (ed) Diseases of the Breast 1996].
[Kopans DB, 15th Ann Int Miami Breast Cancer Conf: February 26–28, 1998].
[Kopans DB, Cancer Supplement, 72(4): 1457–1460, 1993].
[Kopans DB, Breast Imaging, Philadelphia, JB Lippincott, 1998].

- The standard screening modalities are mammogram and physical examination and they are complementary.
  – Mammogram can detect cancer earlier than any other modality.

- Mammography is the only technique with proven efficacy for breast cancer screening.

- Mammographically discovered lesions average < 0.5 cm in diameter and are therefore less likely to be metastatic.
  – Most mammographically detected lesions should be ≤ 1.5 cm in diameter.

- Several Randomized controlled studies have confirmed that mammographic screening of asymptomatic ♀ plus regular physical examinations reduce the death rate from breast cancer by 20–30% in ♀ > 50 years old [Tabár L, Radiology Clinics of North America 30: 187–210, 1992].

- With the exception of two studies, most trials have shown a 20–30% reduction in breast cancer related mortality for ♀ age 50–65 years who undergo mammography compared to those who do not.

- Based on the Surveillance, Epidemiology, and End Results (SEER) program of the NCI estimates, in 1993 alone, 28 900 women, age 40–49, were diagnosed with breast cancer. This was only 8% fewer than the number of women who were diagnosed between the ages of 50–59 (31 500).

- Recent data from the Gothenburg Screening Trial show a 45% reduction in mortality for screened ♀ age 40–49. [Bjurstam N, Cancer 80(11): 2091–2099, 1997].

- Important to emphasize that all Randomized controlled trials involve mammography of the 1980's or earlier; results with state-of-the-art mammography should be better.

- More than 40% of the years of life lost to breast cancer occur in ♀ d before the age of 50.

- There is no significant difference in the mammographic image of breast tissue in women ages 40–49 compared to women ages 50–59. The breasts do not turn to fat at the moment of menopause or at age 50.
  - There is ↑ breast fat content with age, but this is gradual.

Randomized controlled mammography trials				
Trial	Intervention arm vs. control arm	No. of subjects	Age groups (years)	Percentage reduction in cancer mortality
Health Insurance Plan of NY [1]	Mammogram (M) + Physical examination (PE) yearly ×4	62 000	40–64 60–64	23 21
Two-county trial in Sweden [2]	M q 24–33 months	163 000	40–74 50–69	31 39
UK [3]	M biennially x 7 PE yearly x 7	237 000	45–64	24
Malmö Trial [4] (Sweden)	M q 18–24 months	42 000	45–69 55–69	4 20
Canadian National Breast Cancer Screening Study [5]	M + PE yearly × 5	89 835	40–49 50–60	NR 3
Gothenburg Breast Cancer Screening Trial (6)	M q 18 mo	25 941	39–49	45
[1] Schapiro S, J Natl Cancer Inst 69: 349–55, 1982. [2] Tabár L. Lancet 339: 412–4, 1992. [3] UK Trial, Lancet 2: 411–6, 1988. [4] Anderson I, Br Med J 297: 943–8, 1988. [5] Miller AB, Can Med Assoc J. 147: 1459–88, 1992. [6] Bjurstam N, Cancer 80(11): 2091–2099, 1997.				

- Limitations of the Canadian study:
  - Randomization flawed.
  - Contamination of both groups.

- 26% of control group (unscreened), had mammograms done privately.
- Poor quality mammography and interpretation.

● Low level radiation from modern mammograms has not been shown to be carcinogenic.

● The debate among physicians is whether to start screening at age 40 or 50.

● Mammography every 1–2 years saves lives in ♀ older than 50. It has not been shown to save lives in ♀ less than 50 years old, until the recent report of the Swedish Two-County Trial, listed below. Trends exist and multiple reasons related to both study design and biology of breast cancer that have led to negative studies.

● The studies to date were not designed to look at different age groups and too few ♀ age 40–49 were evaluated to provide clear evidence of difference in mortality.
[Fletcher SW, J Natl Cancer Inst 85: 1644–1656, 1993].
- 8 Randomized controlled trials have evaluated ∼ 167 000 ♀, ages 40–49. One would need ∼ 500 000 ♀ to show a statistically significant decrease in mortality of 25–30%.
- Also the duration most of the studies has not been long enough to show significance in this younger age group.

● [Tabár L, Breast Cancer Res Treat 46(1), 1997].
- The Swedish Two-County Trial produced data to support annual mammographic screening in ♀ age 40–49.
- Mean follow-up 16 years.
- Conducted from 1977–1985.
- 133 000 ♀ ages 40–75 years.
- Half of the ♀ were 'invited' to undergo regular mammography; half were not.
- Overall, the trial showed a 42% reduction in the relative risk for breast cancer mortality in the screened group.
- Data showed that the progression from preclinical to clinical cancer varies by age.
  - Younger ♀ progressed more rapidly than older ♀.
- Data also indicated that small preclinical, mammographically detectable breast cancers are just as likely to be low grade in younger ♀ as in older ♀, and therefore just as likely to be curable.

Official recommendations for screening by the American College of Radiology and the American Cancer Society, and other organizations. [American Cancer Society, Workshop on [American Cancer Society, Workshop on Guidelines for Breast Cancer Detection. Chicago, March 7–9, 1997]; [NCI, National Cancer Advisory Board issues mammography screening recommendations. NIH, March 27, 1997]; [Dodd GD Cancer 69: 1885–1887, 1992].

- Bilateral mammograms.
  - By age 40: baseline mammogram.
  - Age 40–49: every 1–2 years.
    - Accompanied by physical examination.
  - Age ≥ 50: every year.
    - Accompanied by physical examination.
  - No upper age limit.

- Self examination.
  - 7–10% of palpable masses are not seen on mammograms.
  - Premenopausal ♀.
    - 5–7 days after their menstrual period every month.
  - Postmenopausal ♀.
    - Same day every month.

- Clinical breast examination by physician.
  - American Cancer Society recommendations:
    - Age 20–40.
      - Examination by physician q 3 years.
    - Age ≥ 40.
      - Examination by physician q 2–3 years.

- Tumor markers.
  - Currently not recommended as screening tests.

Screening mammography

- Definition: the process of finding abnormalities that may be breast cancer.
  - Purpose: detect early breast cancer.
  - Performed on asymptomatic ♀.
  - Two routine films (craniocaudal and medial lateral oblique).

— The entire breast is not imaged.
— Physician presence not required.
— Read as normal or abnormal.

Diagnostic mammography

● Definition: the process of determining which of the abnormalities is actually breast cancer.
— Performed on symptomatic ♀.
— Tailored to specific problem.
— Physician is present.
— Indications for asymptomatic ♀.
  — ♀ with abnormality detected at screening.
  — Follow-up study.
  — Breast cancer follow-up.
  — Status post augmentation mammoplasty.

● Functions:
1. Identify palpable and nonpalpable lesions.
2. Define extent of lesion (tumor size).
3. Locate tumor.
4. Determine need for re-excision.
   — After biopsy → repeat unilateral mammogram with magnification to make sure there is no residual nonpalpable disease because the margins are not always accurate.
   — Wait 2–3 weeks for edema to resolve.

● There are no absolute mammographic criteria which distinguish malignant from benign lesions.

● It is important to determine whether calcifications are truly intramammary or in the skin.

● Morphology and distribution are the most important elements in the analysis of calcifications.

● Magnification mammography is the primary technique to use to further analyze calcifications.

● Calcifications that vary in size and shape are suspicious for malignancy.

- Mammographic findings consistent with benign breast disease:
  - Solid or lucent centered spheres.
  - Smooth, round calcifications with lucent centers.
  - > 1 mm in diameter.
  - The presence of large calcifications (> 0.5 mm) in a mass make it more likely to be a benign lesion such as an involuting fibroadenoma or papilloma.
  - Sedimented calcium settles to the bottom of cysts (milk of calcium).
  - Vascular calcifications.
    - Have a distinctive parallel track appearance.

- Mammographic findings suspicious for malignancy:
  1. Irregular or spiculated mass.
  2. Clustered microcalcifications (could be benign).
     - Biopsy is needed to establish accurate diagnosis.
  3. Most of the calcifications associated with breast cancer are < 0.5 mm in diameter.
  4. Solid nodule with ill-defined borders.
  5. Architectural distortion.
  6. Enlarging solid, well-circumscribed mass.
  7. Developing density-compared with previous films.
  8. Focal asymmetric density.

- The sine qua non of breast cancer **is a high attenuation mass with spiculated margins**.
  - The spicules represent fibrous reaction to the malignant lesion.
    - Tumor may or may not extend along the spicules.
    - Spiculated abnormality: differential diagnosis.
      1. Malignancy.
      2. Malignancy.
      3. Malignancy.
      4. Post surgical or radial scar (benign).
      5. Area of fat necrosis.

  - Negative mammogram in the setting of a breast mass requires evaluation to rule out malignancy.

  - Mammography has a false negative rate of ~ 10–30%.
    - Biopsy should be performed for all palpable lesions.
    - Mammography cannot be used to exclude breast cancer.

— Reasons for false negatives.
1. Mass hides within dense breast tissue (most common reason).
2. Screening mammogram does not include all of the breast.
3. Infiltrating lobular carcinoma (very difficult to image).
4. Poor quality study.
5. Interpretation error.

- 3% of normal ♀ have asymmetric breast tissue without evidence of architectural distortion on mammogram or palpable mass.
  - Mammography after needle biopsy.
    — It is always better to obtain the mammogram prior to any intervention.
    — After needle biopsy it is advised to wait two weeks or more after the procedure is completed so that tissue changes can resolve.

- Mammographic changes after surgery.
  — Focal skin thickening and retraction at surgical site.
  — Variable amount of distortion and/or mass at the tumor bed.

- Mammographic changes after XRT.
  — Edema: usually distributed in the gravity affected portions of the breast, i.e. periareolar, inferiorly and medially.
  — Coarse trabecular changes.
  — Egg shell type calcifications (calcium around areas of liquified fat, i.e. fat necrosis).
  — Early calcifications of fat necrosis may be indistinguishable from malignancy.
  — Oil cysts.

- Use of mammogram post surgery + XRT.
  — To evaluate for new mass/calcifications.
  — Obtain a new baseline mammogram 6 months after the completion of XRT.
  — For further details, please refer to the section: 'Following Breast Cancer Patients' on page 154.

IMAGING STUDIES
[Kopans DB and Rubin E, 15th Ann Int Miami Breast Cancer Conf: February 26–28, 1998].
[Kopans DB, Cancer Supplement, 72(4): 1457–1460, 1993].
[Kopans DB, Breast Imaging, Philadelphia, JB Lippincott, 1998].

Ultrasound (USN)

- It is the most operator dependent of all imaging modalities.

- Not for screening.

- Guided by physical examination or mammogram to determine if the lesion already detected is cystic or solid.

MRI

- Highly sensitive.
  - Leads to an unnecessary number of biopsies.

- Currently investigational for screening and staging.

- Does not visualize calcifications.

- Since it reflects tumor vascularity, it may be beneficial in differentiating post surgical scar vs. local recurrence.
  - Studies ongoing.

- Imaging method of choice verifying the integrity of implants.

- More sensitive than bone scan to detect bone metastases, if there is suspicion.

Bone scan

- Good screening test for detection of metastases in asymptomatic ♀ with stage III breast cancer.
  - Bone metastases detected in 20–25% of these ♀.

- Not good for screening ♀ with stage I/II breast cancer.
  - Bone metastases detected in < 5% of these ♀.

PET scan

- Currently being studied.

Sestamibi scan

- Under advanced evaluation.

Liver scan

- Not for screening.
  - Reserve for patients with abnormal liver chemistry and hepatomegaly.
  - Histologic confirmation is often necessary.
  - Almost completely displaced by CT scan and ultrasound.

EVALUATION OF A PALPABLE BREAST MASS AND NIPPLE DISCHARGE

[Donegan WL, New Engl J Med 327(13): 937–942, 1992].

History and physical examination

- In the past breast cancer most commonly presented as a palpable mass and was usually found by the patient.
  - In the U.S. today, most breast cancers are detected mammographically.

- Suggestive of malignant mass.
  - Hard, painless mass.
  - May be fixed to chest wall or skin.
  - Dimpling of skin (Fig. 3).
  - Retraction of nipple.
  - Bloody discharge.
  - Masses in irradiated breasts of ♀ treated by lumpectomy are especially suspicious.

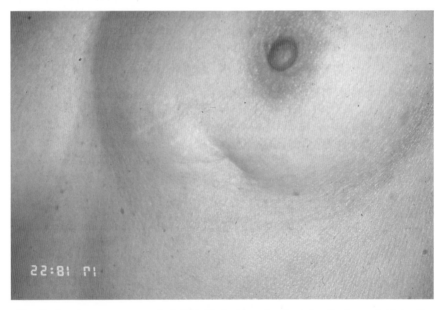

Fig. 3. Spontaneous or provoked (dimpling) skin retraction should always lead to the suspicion of breast cancer even if there is nothing palpable.

- Suggestive of benign mass.
  - Firm, rubbery mass.
  - $\pm$ Pain: breast cancer can be painful $\sim 10\%$ of the cases.
  - Discrete regular margins.
  - Mobile.

- Cysts cannot be distinguished from solid masses reliably by physical examination.

- Nipple discharge.
  - Suspicious features.
    - Unilateral from one duct orifice.
    - Spontaneous.
  - Test for occult blood.
  - Note color and consistency.
    - Serous, serosanguineous, bloody (red, brown or black) and clear colorless discharge should be investigated further.
    - Milky discharge from multiple ducts or bilaterally is usually hormonal or related to medication.
    - Thick green, yellow or brown discharge is usually associated with duct ectasia and most often is a non-spontaneous discharge from multiple orifices bilaterally.
    - Galactography
      - May help identify the cause of the discharge and the location of the lesion.
      - Benefit is controversial.

  - LDH isoenzyme assay of nipple discharge: may be useful in diagnosis of breast cancer. [Kawamoto M, Cancer 73: 1836–1841, 1994].

Needle aspiration

- Safe, simple and inexpensive.

- Immediately distinguishes cysts from solid masses.

- Cysts.
  - Frequent cause of masses in perimenopausal ♀.
  - ↑ frequency as menopause approaches.
    - Cytology: only submit bloody fluid.
      [Ciatto S, Acta Cytol 31:301–304, 1987].
      - Ciatto et al. found no malignancy in 6747 nonbloody specimens.

— Simple cyst aspiration.
  — Typically the fluid is not bloody.
  — Mass disappears after aspiration (leaving temporary defect).
  — Mammogram is normal after aspiration.
— Intracystic carcinoma or partially cystic cancers: ↑ suspicion.
  — Bloody aspirate.
  — Palpable mass remains after all fluid is withdrawn.
  — Cyst repeatedly refills (< 9% of simple cysts will refill after 2–3 aspirations).
  — Mammographic density persists after aspiration.

● Solid mass.
  — Suggested by failure to aspirate cystic fluid.
  — Indication for FNA and cytologic examination.
  — FNA will not determine invasiveness of tumor.
  — Needle core biopsy (NCB) is more accurate than FNA in establishing diagnosis.

Mammography

● Purpose of mammography.
  — Characterize mass.
  — Detect clinically occult lesions.
    — Bilateral simultaneous cancers are reported in 1–3% of cases; a majority of these are found with mammography.

● Candidates for mammography.
  — All patients with breast mass, even when cancer is obvious.
  — Exception:
    — ♀ < 20 years old.
      — Risk of a single mammogram at young age is still low.

    — Pregnancy.
      — In ♀ with known breast cancer or highly suspicious finding during pregnancy or lactation, a mammogram should be performed.

● Radiation risk of mammography
  — Mean glandular dose (MGD) is a preferred unit of measure for dose from mammography.
  — The American College of Radiology (ACR) recommends for a 4.5 cm thick breast:
    — 3 m Gy (300 m rad) for film/screen with grid; which is the usual.
    — 1 mGy (100 m rad) for film/screen without grid.

— Radiation-induced breast cancers.
  — Result from MGDs in 1–20 Gy range (100–2000 rad).
    — As they occurred in atom bomb survivors, tuberculosis patients with repeated fluoroscopies, and radiation therapy patients.
  — Little data is available for MGD < 0.5 Gy (50 rad).
    — Still nearly 200 × higher than the dose risk for a single mammogram.
  — Extrapolation from available data suggests two excess breast cancer deaths might result from exposing one million ♀, 45 years of age and older, to MGD of 1 m Gy (100 m rad).
    — 1500 expected breast cancer cases in 1 million ♀.
    — Case fatality in absence of screening ∼ 50%.
    — Screening program reduces mortality by ∼ 40% or 300 lives saved.
  — Risk:benefit.
    — 300:2.

Ultrasound

● Distinguishes solid from cystic mass.

● In adolescent women, often is the only imaging study needed.

● Needle aspiration is superior to ultrasound.
  — Quicker.
  — Less expensive.
  — Equally accurate.
  — Provides therapeutic relief for cysts.

CT/MRI/MRI

● No established place in evaluation.

● Both can distinguish cystic from solid masses, but aspiration and sonography are quicker and cheaper.

Open biopsy

● Core biopsy of a palpable breast mass or stereotactic biopsy of a non-palpable mass, wherever available, are accurate for definitive diagnosis in the majority of patients.

● Some masses still require an open biopsy for definitive diagnosis.

BREAST PATHOLOGY
[Tavassoli FA, Pathology of the Breast, Elsevier, 1992].
[Harris JR, New Engl J Med 327(6): 390–398, 1992].

- Two comparable grading systems currently used are:
  1. NSABP, Dr Fisher's method [Fisher ER, Pathol Ann 15: 239–251, 1980].
     — Combines nuclear grade, histologic grade and mitoses.
  2. Scarff-Bloom-Richardson (SBR) Classification
     [Bloom HJG, Br J Cancer 11: 359–377, 1957]
     [Scarff RW, Geneva, WHO 2: 13–18, 1968].
     — Scores the combination of tubule formation, nuclear pleomorphism and mitotic rate.
     — 3–5 points → grade I (well differentiated).
     — 6–7 points → grade II (moderately differentiated).
     — 8–9 points → grade III (poorly differentiated).

- Histologic (tissue) grade
  — How much tumor looks like ductal structures (ducts).
    I. Ducts present: > 75% (well differentiated).
    II. Ducts present: 10–75% (moderately differentiated).
    III. Ducts present: < 10% (poorly differentiated).

- Nuclear grade:
  — Depends on:
    — Size of nucleus.
    — Density of stain (the darker the stain, the more DNA).
    — Variation of shape.
  — Grade I: uniformly staining nucleus; best prognosis.
  — Grade II/III: worst prognosis.

- Mitoses.
  — Low $0-3.3/mm^2$
  — Medium $3.3-7/mm^2$
  — High $>7/mm^2$

Important to distinguish:

- Multifocality [Holland R, Cancer 56: 979–90, 1985].
  — Definition:
    — Two or more foci of cancer, < 5 cm apart in the same breast.
  — Common, and can be extensive.

- Multicentricity.
  - Definition:
    - Two or more foci of cancer, > 5 cm apart in the same breast.
    - Usually means lesions are in different quadrants.
  - Frequency: ~ 25% of cancers.
  - Clinical multicentricity is rare.
  - Multicentric disease has been associated with:
    - Large primary tumor size (≥ 5 cm).
    - Centrally located tumors.
    - Invasive lobular cancer.
    - EIC (extensive intraductal component).
    - LN (+).

- Nijmegen (Netherlands) Trial.
  [Holland R, 15th International Miami Breast Cancer Conference, February 26–28, 1998].
  - > 2000 mastectomy specimens evaluated.
  - Multicentricity < 10%.
  - Multifocality was the more common, with ~ 60%.

- Bilaterality.
  - Patients at ↑ risk of contralateral breast cancer:
    - Young age.
    - Nipple involvement.
    - Size of mass > 2 cm.
    - Lobular histology.
  - Incidence ↓ after menopause.
  - 1% per year rate of developing cancer in the opposite breast.
  - High quality mammogram of contralateral breast is necessary.
  - Blinded mirror image contralateral biopsy has no role.

Non-invasive breast cancer

- Ductal carcinoma *In Situ* (DCIS).
  - Proliferation of cancerous cells within the ducts.
  - It is a morphologic marker of risk.
    - A biopsy (+) for DCIS ↑ the risk of subsequently developing infiltrating ductal breast carcinoma, 8–10 × ; and this risk may be higher in comedo DCIS. [Ward BA, Arch Surg 127: 1392–1395, 1992].

— There is no germline mutation.
  — Allelic deletion or loss of heterozygosity (LOH) has been widely reported in DCIS. [Stratton M, J Pathol 175: 195–201, 1995].
— Thought to be precursor of invasive ductal carcinoma.
— Heterogeneous:
  — 1. Extent of involvement.
  — 2. Nuclear grade.
— DCIS at times may be difficult to differentiate cytologically and architecturally from atypical ductal hyperplasia.
— Often detected by mammogram as microcalcifications.
— The distribution of DCIS is usually segmental and grows toward the nipple.
  — Biopsies should be done by the surgeon in the shape of a cone and toward the nipple.
  — Samples should be marked with ink toward the direction of the nipple.
  — Samples should be sectioned by the pathologist toward the direction of the nipple.
— Poorly differentiated (high grade) DCIS most of the time is continuous.
— Well differentiated (low grade) DCIS most of the time is multifocal, not continuous.

— Categories:

  1. Comedo.
     — Always with necrosis and almost always with high nuclear grade.
     — Mitoses are often numerous.
     — ~ 80% of Comedo lesions are aneuploid, ER (−), and have a high rate of c-erbB-2 overexpression.
     — Worst prognosis.
     — Higher rate of local recurrence.

  2. Non-comedo.
     — Mitoses are relatively infrequent.
     a. Cribriform → best prognosis.
     b. Micropapillary.
     c. Papillary.
     d. Solid.

  3. Comedo and non-comedo DCIS as well as LCIS may all coexist within the same breast.

- DCIS vs Invasive breast cancer
  - FNA cannot reliably distinguish DCIS from invasive carcinoma.
  - Frozen section has no role in evaluating nonpalpable, mammographically detected focus of microcalcification or its margins intraoperatively.
  - This approach limits the ability of pathologists to evaluate lesion.
  - Histologically, the main difference between DCIS and infiltrating carcinoma is the way DCIS preserves the ductal/lobular anatomy. Unlike DCIS, infiltrative carcinoma forms structures not usually present, such as strands of epithelium and nodules.
  - One difference between invasive breast cancer and intraductal breast cancer may be that intraductal breast cancer cells make their own basement membrane.
  - Point of interest: retinoic acid is a regulator of basement membrane synthesis and it is being studied, along with some of its derivatives, in chemoprevention trials.

- Lobular carcinoma *In Situ* (LCIS).
  - Uniform solid proliferation of small cells within multiple breast lobules, and occasionally in ducts with small, uniform nuclei and distinct cell borders; leading to dilatation of the involved acini of the lobules and the loss of cohesion.
  - Commonly multicentric.
  - Risk of ipsilateral breast cancer → 10–17%.
  - Risk of contralateral breast cancer → 10–25%.
  - Up to 37% of the patient with known LCIS in one breast will eventually develop invasive cancer if both breasts are left intact.
    - Equal frequency in either breast.
  - Often shows a gradual continuum of atypia.
    - Lobular neoplasia (LN1), (LN2) and (LN3 = LCIS).
    - LN1 and LN2 often called atypical lobular hyperplasia.
    - LN2-the outline of the acini is maintained.
    - LN3 (LCIS)-there is so much distention of the acini, that it appears confluent.
  - LCIS and atypical lobular hyperplasia (ALH):
    - The type and degree of epithelial proliferation within the lobules distinguishes ALH and LCIS.
    - Both are at ↑ risk of developing breast cancer.
    - Subsequent development of carcinoma is nine times greater in patients with LCIS than in patients with ALH.

- LCIS lacks clinical or mammographic signs.
- Difficult to diagnose by mammography.
  - Tends not to calcify and often has indefinite margins.
- Surgical (−) margins not required, since it is presumed to be multicentric.
- Frozen sections are not reliable, because there is no palpable tumor.

Microinvasive breast cancer

- Can be seen in association with DCIS and LCIS.

- It is the first stage in the development of invasion.

- It was found in < 1% of all breast cancers reviewed at the Armed Forces Institute of Pathology (AFIP).

- Controversial data because it is very rare.
  [Silver S, Cancer 82: 2382–2390 1998].
  - 38 cases retrospectively reviewed at AFIP.
    - 29 ♀ with DCIS and microinvasion.
    - 9 ♀ with DCIS with probable microinvasion.
  - Mean age: 56 years.
  - Treatment: mastectomy with axillary LN dissection.
  - Microinvasion was defined as invasive carcinoma ≤ 2 mm or < 3 foci of invasion each ≤ 1 mm in maximum diameter.
  - Mean number of LNs resected → 19. (range, 7–38 LNs).
  - Mean follow-up → 7.5 years (range, 1–14.4 years).
  - Nodal status → all axillary LNs resected were negative.
  - None of the 33 patients followed for a mean of 7.5 years developed a local recurrence or metastases.
  - Conclusion:
    - Microinvasion defined as invasive carcinoma ≤ 2 mm or < 3 foci of invasion each ≤ 1 mm in size in maximum diameter, is not associated with LN invasion and has an excellent prognosis.

Invasive breast cancer

1. Infiltrating ductal carcinoma (invasive ductal carcinoma)
   - Most common breast carcinoma (~ 75%).
   - Microscopically characterized by being variably thick strands (> 1 cell layer), often with tubule formation, usually grade II/III nuclei, sometimes solid tumor nodules, central sclerosis, necrosis, often with DCIS.

— Characterized by stony hardness at palpation.
— Gritty resistance is encountered upon transection; used to be called 'scirrhous' carcinoma.
  [Carter D, Am J Surg Pathol 2: 39–46, 1978].
— Tumors with stellate configuration and focal necrosis have an especially poor prognosis.
— More frequently metastasizes to bone, lung and liver.

2. Infiltrating lobular carcinoma.
  — ~ 5–10% of breast cancer.
  — Characterized by ill-defined thickening or induration in the breast.
    — Can be difficult to identify grossly.
    — Frequently presents in the upper outer quadrant.
  — Microscopically, composed of small cells in a linear arrangement 'Indian File' with tendency to grow around ducts and lobules.
  — Greater proportion of multicentric tumors, either in the same or opposite breast, compared to infiltrating ductal carcinoma.
  — More often metastasizes to meninges (carcinomatous meningitis), serosal surfaces, ovaries and retroperitoneum.
    — Intestinal and ureteral obstruction can occur.

3. Tubular carcinoma.
  — Also known as well-differentiated carcinoma.
  — ~ 2% of all breast cancer.
  — ≥ 75% of tumors composed of simple, well-formed tubules lined by single layers of cells.
  — Low nuclear grade.
  — Axillary metastases are rare.
  — Better prognosis than infiltrating ductal carcinoma.
  — Can be difficult to distinguish from radial scar (benign proliferative lesion).
  — Typically ER(+) and PR(+).

4. Medullary carcinoma.
  — ~ 5–7% of all breast cancer.
  — ♀ tend to be younger at diagnosis (< 50 years old).
  — Axillary LN tend to be large, even in the absence of nodal metastases.
  — Characterized microscopically by sheets of tumor (not strands), poorly differentiated nuclei, intense infiltration of small lymphocytes (mostly T-lymphocytes) and plasma cells, well-circumscribed border and little or no associated DCIS.

— Better prognosis than infiltrating ductal carcinoma.
— Must have all above features for better prognosis.
  — 'Atypical' medullary carcinoma has some features of medullary, but has the same prognosis as infiltrating ductal carcinoma.
— Typically ER(−) and PR(−).
— Frequently (−) membrane immunoreactivity for HER2/neu oncogene.
— Usually (+) nuclear immunoreactivity for p53, indicating p53 mutation.

5. Mucinous or colloid carcinoma.
   — 3% of all breast cancer.
   — Characterized by abundant accumulation of extracellular mucin around clusters of tumor cells.
   — It is slow growing and can become bulky.
   — When the tumor is predominantly mucinous the prognosis tends to be favorable.
   — Pure mucinous carcinomas usually are diploid whereas most mixed mucinous tumors tend to be aneuploid.
   — Unusual complication:
     — Cerebral infarction due to mucin embolism.

6. Papillary carcinoma.
   — ~ 1–2% of all breast cancer.
   — Tends to occur in older ♀.
   — Mostly a variant of an in situ cancer.
   — Tumor lines fibrous stalks.
   — Lacks myoepithelial cells.
   — Often diffuse (multifocal).
   — Good prognosis.
   — Typically ER(+).

● The following types: pure colloid, tubular, papillary, medullary are commonly felt to have a lower incidence of nodal involvement and a better prognosis for any given tumor size.

● Other rare carcinomas include: apocrine, squamous cell carcinoma, spindle cell carcinoma, carcinosarcoma and Merkle-cell carcinoma.

● Paget disease.
   — Intraepidermal adenocarcinoma of nipple.
   — Neoplastic eczematoid changes around the nipple.

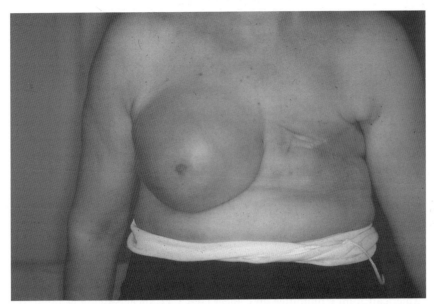

Fig. 4. Carcinomatose mastitis. Diffuse inflammation of the breast without a palpable nodule may be malignant, especially if there is a history of contralateral breast cancer.

— Clinically appears as a rash on the nipple.
  — Almost always associated with underlying ductal carcinoma
  — For more details, refer to Unusual Presentations, page 159.

- Inflammatory breast carcinoma.
  — Most aggressive.

  — ~ 1% of breast cancer in USA.

  — ~ 25% of these patients have breast or nipple pain.

— Rapid onset.
  — It is a clinical and/or pathological diagnosis:
  — Marked by diffuse erythema and brawny induration of the skin of the breast, sometimes with a peau d'orange (skin of an orange) appearance and tumor cell emboli that plug the dermal lymphatics (Fig. 4).
  — Biopsy → Infiltrating breast cancer that classically has dermal lymphatic invasion (with or without lymphatic invasion, prognosis is the same).
  — Mammogram may show skin edema.

— Primary stage IIIb breast cancer.

— It is treated as other types of stage III disease, but the prognosis is worse if untreated.
  — Combined modalities are a must!

— 90% probability of axillary LN involvement.

— 25–50% of all patients develop contralateral breast cancer.
  — Usually in the setting of metastatic disease.

— Typically ER(−) and PR(−).

— Common in Northern Africa (Tunisia) where it is associated with pregnancy or lactation.

STAGING

[Manual for Staging of Cancer, 4th Ed. OH Beahrs (Ed) JB Lippincott, pp 149–154, 1992].
[American Joint Committee on Cancer (AJCC) Cancer Staging Manual, ID Fleming (Ed)
Lippincott-Raven, pp 171–180, 1997].

TNM system

● Surgical staging system.

Size

● T_x Pimary tumor cannot be assessed.

● T_0 No evidence of primary tumor.

● T_{is} Carcinoma in situ: intraductal carcinoma, lobular carcinoma in situ, or Paget's disease of the nipple with no tumor.

● T_1 < 2 cm.
  a. Tumor ≤ 0.5 cm.
  b. Tumor > 0.5 cm, and ≤ 1 cm.
  c. Tumor > 1 cm, and ≤ 2 cm.

● T_2 2–5 cm.

● T_3 > 5 cm.

- T_4 Any size tumor with extension into the chest wall or skin.
  a. Extension to chest wall.
  b. Edema (including peau d'orange), ulceration of the skin of the breast, or satellite skin nodules confined to the same breast.
  c. Both of the above.
  d. Inflammatory carcinoma.

Nodes

- N_x Regional LN cannot be assessed.

- N_0 No nodes.

- N_1 (+) moveable, ipsilateral axillary nodes.

- N_2 Fixed or matted ipsilateral axillary nodes.

- N_3 Ipsilateral internal mammary nodes.

Metastases

- M_x Distant metastases cannot be assessed.

- M_0 No metastases.

- M_1 Metasases.

Clinical staging

- Stage 0
  — Intraductal cancer (ductal carcinoma in situ).

- Stage I
  — Small tumor, no nodal involvement.
  — < 2 cm, (−)LN
  — Refers only to $T_1N_0M_0$.

- Stage II
  — 2–5 cm.
  — (+)LN in axilla, no matted nodes.

- Stage III
  — Locally advanced disease.
  — Any tumor matted or skin changes.
  — > 5 cm, (+) Internal mammary LN, metastases to skin (inflammatory).

Stage	TNM Grouping
0	$T_{is} N_0 M_0$
I	$T_1 N_0 M_0$
IIA	$T_0 N_1 M_0$ $T_0 N_1^* M_0$ $T2 N_0 M_0$
IB	$T_2 N_1 M_0$ $T_3 N_0 M_0$
IIIA	$T_0 N_2 M_0$ $T_1 N_2 M_0$ $T_2 N_2 M_0$ $T_3 N_1 M_0$ $T_3 N_2 M_0$
IIIB	T_4 any N M_0 Any T, $N_3 M_0$
IV	Any T, any N, M_1

* The prognosis of patients with stage N_{1_a} disease is similar to that of patients with stage N_0 disease

— Stage IIIA
  — Locally advanced non-metastatic (M_0) breast cancer that is technically operable.
  — T > 5 cm and palpable axillary LN.
  — Tumor of any size with fixed axillary nodes.
— Stage IIIB
  — Tumor of any size that extends to the chest wall or skin (T_4) or metastases to the ipsilateral internal mammary LN chain (N_3).
  — Inoperable by virtue of low probability of obtaining clear surgical margins.

● Stage IV
  — Distant metastases.
  — Invasion of primary into chest wall and if there is an adjacent nodule invading the chest wall.
— Chest wall recurrence (relapse).

—Ipsilateral supraclavicular node involvement.
—Internal mammary node involvement.

Survival

[American Joint Committee for Cancer Staging and End Results, 1983].
[American Joint Committee on Cancer (AJCC) Cancer Staging Manual, ID Fleming (Ed) Lippincott-Raven, 1997].

	Overall survival	
TNM Stage	5 year survival (%)	10 year survival (%)
Stage I	87	78
Stage II	68	52
Stage III	41	28
Stage IV	10	0

PROGNOSTIC FACTORS
[McGuire WL, New Engl J Med 326: 1756–1761, 1992].
[Wong WW, Am J Med 92: 539–548, 1992].

● Primary prognostic factors: nodal status, tumor size, tumor grade,
  and hormone receptor (HR) status.
  1. Lymph node status [Turner-Warwick RT, Br J Surg 46: 574–582,
  1959].
    — 1/4th of the lymphatic drainage of the breast is through the
      ipsilateral internal mammary (IM) nodes and it is from all
      quadrants of the breast.
    [Morrow M, Arch Surg 116: 748–751, 1981].
    — Metastases of the IM nodes in the absence of axillary LN
      involvement is a rare occurrence ($\sim 5\%$).
    — For this reason the extended radical mastectomy, which
      included resection of the IM nodes, was abandoned.
  — The axilla is the principal drainage site for the breast.
  — The number of axillary (+)LNs is the most significant
    prognostic factor.
    — Patients with 1–3 (+) axillary LNs do the best among those
      patients with (+) axillary LNs.

Axillary lymph node prognosis.		
No. of (+) lymph nodes	Recurrence at 5 years (%)	10-year survival (%)
0	~ 20	65–80
1–3	30–40	35–65
4	~ 44	–
>4	~ 54–82	13–24
[Valagussa P, Cancer 41: 1170–1178, 1978].		

[Friedman S, Acta Oncol 27: 483–487, 1988].
[Rosen PP, Ann Surg 194: 585–591, 1981].
  — Significance of histologically determined axillary micrometastases
    (< 0.2 cm) is unknown.
[De Mascarel, Br J Cancer 66: 523–527, 1992].

— Significance of immunohistochemically-determined axillary micrometastases.
  — Using monoclonal antibodies can detect 10–20% of cases of invasive ductal carcinoma thought to be node negative by standard histology.
  — In the group of patients with invasive lobular carcinoma no prognostic value was found, with a median follow-up of 9.3 years.
  — In the group of patients with invasive ductal carcinoma involvement was associated with a statistically significant ↓ in relapse-free survival and overall survival with a median follow-up of 15.6 years.

2. Tumor size.
— Tumor size has (+) correlation with odds of nodal involvement.

Tumor size (cm)	Percentage of axillary nodal involvement (%)
< 1	< 20–30
1–2 cm	27–39
2–3	29–57

— Infiltrating ductal or lobular lesions < 1 cm correlate with good prognosis
  [Rosen PP, J Clin Oncol 11: 2090–2100, 1993].
— Memorial series followed for more than two decades after definitive surgery.
— 767 breast cancer patients.
— Staging at surgery = T_1/T_2, LN(−).
— Neither adjuvant radiation nor chemotherapy were employed.
— Patients with infiltrating ductal or lobular lesions less than or equal to 1 cm in diameter had an 88% chance of no recurrence in 20 years (12% relapse rate at 20 years).

3. Hormone receptor (HR) status.
  — ER/PR(+) → improved prognosis.
  — ER(+) tumors respond to endocrine therapy in ~ 60% of patients.

— The exogenous use of estrogens may mask the estrogen receptor by occupying all binding sites, leading to a false negative result on steroid binding assays of a breast tumor, if a biochemical assay is used, not immunocytochemical.

4. Histopathology.
   [Hopton DS, Eur J Surg Oncol 15: 25–31, 1989].
   [Le D, Cancer 64: 1914–1921, 1989].

Nuclear grade—nuclear staining/anaplasia	
I	Well differentiated, best prognosis
II	Moderately differentiated
III	Porly differentiated, worst prognosis

Histologic grade—degree of tubule formation	
I	Well differentiated, >75% tubule formation, best prognosis
II	Moderately differentiated, 10–75% tubule formation
III	Poorly differentiated, <10% tubule formation, worst prognosis

— Nuclear grade.
  — Indicates degree of differentiation.
  — Grade II, III → worse prognosis.
— Histologic grade.
  — Indicates degree of tubule formation.
  — Grade II,III → worse prognosis.

5. S-phase.
   [Hedley DW, Cytometry 14: 482–485, 1993].
   — Indicates rate of cell proliferation.
   — High S-phase → worse prognosis.
   — Espcially important in LN(−) disease.
   — Becoming an independent prognostic factor.

6. DNA ploidy.
   — Diploid tumors: associated with good prognosis.
   — Significance not clear.

● The Nottingham Prognostic Index (NPI)
   [Kollias J, Br J Cancer 75: 1318–1323, 1997].
   [Blamey RW, 15th Ann Int Miami Breast Cancer Conf, February 26–28, 1998].
   — On multivariate analysis only three factors remained with independent significance.
   — Tumor size.
   — Histologic grade.
   — Lymph node status.
   — The NPI has been tested prospectively among 1168 ♀ in Nottingham and furthermore it has been tested among 9000 ♀ in a series in Denmark.

The NPI	Nottingham (%)	Denmark (%)	10-year survival (%)	
			Nottingham	Denmark
Good	27	29	79	83
Moderate	57	54	56	52
Poor	15	17	24	13

● **New prognostic factors**
   1. HER-2/neu receptor (c-erbB-2 receptor).
      [Winstanley J. Br J Cancer 63: 447–450, 1991].
      [Paterson MC, Cancer Res 51: 556–567, 1991].
      [Ravdin PM, Gene 159(1): 19–27, 1995].
      — Member of the epidermal growth factor receptor (EGFR) family.
      — Located on chromosome 17q21.
      — Transmembrane tyrosine kinase growth factor receptor.
      — Associated with poor prognosis.

      — Overexpressed in breast cancer, usually by amplification.
         — Overexpressed in 16–26% of infiltrating ductal carcinoma.
         [Gusterson BA, J Clin Oncol 10: 1049–1056, 1992].

— Commonly overexpressed in comedo type DCIS (66%).
  [Van de Vijver MJ, New Engl J Med 319: 1239–1245, 1988].

— Overexpressed 10–50% of gastric cancers.

— Not overexpressed by normal cells.

— May be a marker of relative resistance to chemotherapy.
  [Amadori D, Proc Am Soc Clin Oncol 15: 110 (A104) 1996].
  [Head JF, Proc Am Soc Clin Oncol 15: 111 (A108), 1996].

— In the adjuvant setting, some investigators have shown that
  patients with c-erbB-2(+) tumors derive little or no benefit
  from CMF chemotherapy when compared to patients
  receiving no adjuvant chemotherapy. While a recent SWOG
  trial found c-erbB-2(−) tumors do better with CMF
  chemotherapy without deriving benefit from adriamycin
  chemotherapy.

— Important in adriamycin selection and sensitivity.

— CALGB 8869.
  [Muss HB, New Engl J Med 330(18): 1260–1266, 1994].

— 442 LN(+) patients selected from CALGB 8541.

— Subset analysis shows patients that overexpress HER-2/neu
  had an improved overall survival and disease free survival
  with the higher dose of CAF (600/60/600 mg/m^2 q 28 days
  × 4).

— No dose-response relationship was seen in patients with
  primary tumors that had low or absent HER-2/neu
  expression.

— This correlation was not found with S-phase fraction and p53
  accumulation.

— Patients with high c-erbB-2 expression may be more likely to
  respond to taxanes and anthracyclines in the metastatic setting.

— [Carlomagno C, J Clin Oncol 14: 2702–2708, 1996]
  [Leitzel K, J Clin Oncol 13: 1129–1135, 1995]

  — Data from a small series found c-erbB-2(+) tumors resistant
    to tamoxifen while c-erbB-2(−) tumors did well with
    tamoxifen.

    — Large randomized studies need to be done.

[Seidman AD, Proc Am Soc Clin Oncol 15: 104 (A80) 1996].
[Baselga J, J Clin Oncol 14: 737–744, 1996].
- Phase I trials with anti-erb2 antibodies (Herceptin) have shown response in patients that have overexpressed c-erbB-2.
  - For more details, please refer to the Investigational Agents on page 141.

2. p53.
   [Makris A, Lancet 345: 1181–1182, 1995].
   - Located on chromosome 17p13.
   - Normally acts as a tumor-suppressor gene involved in cell cycle regulation.
   - Nuclear protein involved in transcriptional regulation (up and down).
   - Short half-life; therefore cannot be detected in cells.
   - Variety of mutations stabilize the protein resulting in ↑ levels in the cell that are easily detectable.
   - p53 mutations are ubiquitous in human cancers (missense, nonsense, deletion).
   - Expressed in:
     - 50% of metastatic breast cancer with (+) LN.
     - 25% of invasive breast cancer.
     - 13% of intraductal breast cancer.
       [Davidoff AM, J Surg Oncol 48: 260–267, 1991].
     - 20% of comedo DCIS.
   - Not expressed in atypical epithelial hyperplasia or in non-comedo DCIS.
   - There is conflicting data in the literature regarding the prognostic significance of p53 mutations.

3. Epidermal growth factor receptor (EGFR).
   [Fox SB, Breast Cancer Res Treat 29: 41–49, 1994].
   [Nicholson RI, Breast Cancer Res Treat 29: 117–125, 1994].
   - Transmembrane tyrosine kinase receptor.
   - There is a complex family of ligands, often implicated in autocrine loops in breast cancer.
     - Ligand: an extracellular signalling molecule that binds to a specific cell surface receptor.
     - Autocrine loop: tumor cells make the ligand to activate their own receptor in a situation which drives the proliferation of cancer cells.

- Rarely amplified, often overexpressed in breast cancer.
- Associated with poor prognosis.
- Other family members include: c-erbB2/HER2 and HER3 and HER4.
- EGFR(+) tumors are more likely to be resistant to endocrine therapy.
  - Inversely correlated with ER(+).
- Considerable homology with other growth factors/receptors:
  - Insulin receptor.
  - Insulin-like growth factor.
  - Transforming growth factor.

4. Cathepsin D.
   - Thought to be a marker of estrogenic activity.
   - Lysosomal acid protease (aspartyl protease).
   - Believed to be involved in cell surface proteolysis.
   - ↑ levels associated with worse prognosis.
   - [Ravdin PM, J Clin Oncol 12: 467–474, 1994].
     - Cathepsin D was not found to be an independent prognostic factor on multivariate analysis for relapse-free survival among LN(−) ♀ with breast cancer.
   - Other invasion related factors are:
     - Laminin receptor.
     - Angiogenesis factors.

5. Angiogenesis.
   [Griffiths L, Br J Cancer 76: 689–693, 1997].
   [Weidner N, Am J Pathol 147: 9–19, 1995].
   - Angiogenesis plays an important role in the growth and metastases of solid tumors.
   - Activated endothelial cells at the tips of capillaries secrete collagenase, urokinase, and plasminogen activators to allow ingrowth and to facilitate the arrival of oxygen and nutrients to the expanding tumor bed.
   - Intratumoral vascularity (microvessel count).
     - It is a predictor of metastases.
     - On multivariate analysis, it was found to have an independent prognostic significance.
     - Needs to be studied in a prospective randomized manner.

6. Bone marrow micrometastases.

[Vredenburgh JJ, Biology of Blood and Marrow Transplantation 3: 91–97, 1997].

[Vredenburgh JJ, Journal of Hematotherapy 5(1)57–62, 1996].

[Osborne MP, Oncology 8(8): 25–31, 35–36, 39–42, 1994].

[Cote, RJ, J Clin Oncol 9: 1749–1756, 1991].

   — Micrometastases were detected with monoclonal antibodies.
   — Shown to be an independent prognostic factor in several small studies.

[Diel IJ, J Natl Cancer Inst, 88: 1652–1658, 1996].

   — 727 ♀ with primary operable breast cancer from May 1985 to July 1994 were entered into a prospective study.
   — To evaluate the significance of tumor cell detection (TCD) in the bone marrow, also known as bone marrow micrometastases.
   — All ♀ had surgery and axillary LN dissection.
   — Bone marrow aspiration at two sites, on each anterior iliac crest was performed immediately after the surgery.
   — Monoclonal antibody 2E11 directed against the polymorphic epithelial mucin TAG12, was used to detect the tumor cells in the bone marrow samples.
   — Tumor cells were detected in the bone marrow of 203 (55%) of 367 LN(+) ♀ and in 112 (31%) of 360 LN(−) ♀.
   — Tumor cell detection was associated with:
      — Larger tumors ($P < 0.001$).
      — LN involvement ($P = 0.001$).
      — Higher tumor grade ($P = 0.002$).
   — After 36 months of follow-up, ♀ with (+) TCD had both ↓ DFS and ↓ OS (both P-values were < 0.001).
   — TCD was an independent prognostic indicator for both DFS and OS that was superior to axillary LN status, tumor stage, and tumor grade.
   — Among ♀ with tumors < 2 cm in diameter, TCD was the most powerful predictor of outcome.
   — Prospective Randomized trials are needed.

7. Peritumoral lymphatic invasion.

[Gasparini G, J Clin Oncol 12: 454–466, 1994].

   — Peritumoral lymphatic invasion, p53 mutation, and tumor size were found to be independent prognostic factors on multivariate analysis for relapse-free survival among LN(−) ♀ with breast cancer.

[Fisher ER, Cancer 53: 712–723, 1984].
— Peritumoral lymphatic invasion was not an independent prognostic factor of DFS at 10 years in patients who received adjuvant chemotherapy.

8. Perineural invasion.
— Has not been proven to have independent prognostic significance.

9. Obesity.
[Pi-Sunyer FX, Ann Int Med 119: 655–660, 1993].
— A retrospective review of 735 consecutive patients with stage II/III operable primary breast cancer.
— 735 patients with LN(+) primary breast cancer were treated with adjuvant chemotherapy, fluorouracil, doxorubicin, and cyclophosphamide.
— Obesity was defined as 20% above ideal body weight.
— Median follow-up 10.7 years.
— CONCLUSION:
    — The risk of disease recurrence in obese patients was found to be 1.33 times that of non-obese patients.
    — Obesity could be an indicator of poor prognosis for patients with primary breast cancer, even after the administration of adjuvant chemotherapy.

[Zhang S, Cancer 76: 275–283, 1995].
— Correlation between obesity and short disease free survival and overall survival has been reported by other studies.

NON-INVASIVE CANCER

CARCINOMA IN SITU
[Symposium: Contemporary Surgery 49(1): 37–50, 1996].

DCIS

[Silverstein MJ (ed). Ductal Carcinoma In Situ of the Breast. Williams and Wilkins, Baltimore, 1997].
[Schwartz GF, Oncology 8: 21–26, 1994].
[Harris, JR, New Engl J Med 327(6): 390–398, 1992].

- Ductal carcinoma in situ or intraductal breast carcinoma.

- Stage 0.

- 36 400 cases of DCIS in the U.S. in 1997.

- Basement membrane is preserved.

- Seems to arise within the ducts.
  – It is a proliferation of cancerous cells within the ducts <u>without</u> invasion, on light microscopy.

- Typically has a segmental and unicentric distribution, the nipple or subareolar region is commonly involved, and it is often multifocal.
  – Does not invade.
  – Does not cause metastases.

- Mammography has led to earlier detection of non-palpable, subclinical DCIS.
  [Holland R, 15th International Miami Breast Cancer Conference, February 26–28, 1998].
  – Leading to a tremendous ↑ in diagnosis of subclinical DCIS.
  – Mammography usually underestimates the size of DCIS.
  – Microcalcifications are the most common radiographic presentation.
  – Poorly-differentiated DCIS is usually associated with 'casting', coarse-granular microcalcifications which often develop in the necrotic debris of the tumor.

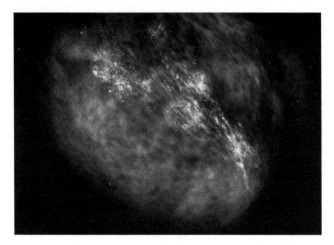

Fig. 5. Typical intraductal distribution of microcalcifications within breast lobe.

- Well-differentiated DCIS is usually associated with fine-granular microcalcifications; these mammographic changes can also be manifested in benign breast lesions (Fig. 5).

• MRI imaging of DCIS leads to too many false(+)s.
  - Still investigational.

• Subtypes of DCIS.
  - For details please refer to PATHOLOGY section.
  - Comedo DCIS and Non-comedo DCIS.

• No systemic chemotherapy is indicated for patients with DCIS.

• The role of tamoxifen in DCIS remains to be defined by the final results of several Randomized trials, such as NSABP-24.

• Mastectomy will cure ∼ 98% of the patients.

• With mastectomy long term studies show 1–2% recurrence rate:
  - [Archer SG, Breast Dis 7: 353–360, 1994].
    - Recurrences occur early in comedo type and late in non-comedo type DCIS.
  - DCIS recurs even after 15 years.

— Half of the recurrent DCIS is <u>invasive</u>.
— Vitrually all of the recurrent DCIS after mastectomy is invasive.

• DCIS cells <u>do not</u> metastasize.

• The goals of breast conserving surgery are:
   — Remove all suspicious microcalcifications.
   — Achieve (−) margins.

Local excision alone
[Lagios MD, Surg Clin North Am 70: 853–871, 1990].
[Lagios MD, The Breast Journal 1: 68–78, 1995].

• Long term studies show:
   — Local recurrence rate 13–60%.
   — 50% of recurrences are invasive.
   — Recurrence rate higher with comedo type vs. non-comedo type.
   — Retrospective results show lumpectomy + XRT decreases recurrence rates compared to excision alone.

• Schwartz Series [Schwartz GF, Ductal Carcinoma in Situ of the Breast (edited by MJ Silverstein) pp 353–360].
   — 191 patients treated with local excision alone.
   — All lesions were 25 mm in diameter or less and found by screening mammogram or incidental biopsy.
   — Clear margins were obtained.
   — Recurrence rate 24.6% at 10 years.
   — Median follow-up: 53 months.

• Lagios series.
   [Lagios MD, Ductal Carcinoma in Situ of the Breast (edited by MJ Silverstein) pp 361–365].
   — 79 ♀ with mammographically detected non-palpable foci of DCIS of histologically confirmed size of 25 mm or less.
   — Lumpectomy only performed without XRT or LN dissection.
   — Median follow-up: 124 months.
   — Overall actuarial local recurrence rate of 19% at 15 years.
   — Half of the recurrences were invasive.
   — Two ♀ with high grade DCIS, (nuclear grade 3) and necrosis developed invasive recurrence with axillary metastases.
      — The second of these ♀ recurred with bilateral invasive breast cancer and axillary metastases after 18 years of follow-up.

- 86% of all recurrences were seen among the high grade DCIS (nuclear grade 3).
- Two recurrences among ♀ with low grade DCIS (nuclear grade 1) were detected mammographically.
  - Both were low grade recurrences in ♀ whose original margins were < 1 mm at the initial excision.
- The most dramatic information obtained retrospectively has been the impact that margin width makes on outcome.
  - 7% local recurrence rate for the widest margin (≥ 1 cm),
        vs.
  - 68% local recurrence rate for the narrowest margin (< 1 mm).
- Local recurrence rate at 15 years,
  - 35% recurrence rate for high grade DCIS (nuclear grade 3)
        vs.
  - 8% recurrence rate for nuclear grade 1 and 2.
- 12/42 ♀ with comedo-type necrosis had a recurrence rate of 29%
        vs.
  3/37 ♀ with no comedo-type necrosis had a recurrence rate of 8%.
- 0/33 patients with DCIS of the micropapillary/non-necrotic cribriform type and low nuclear grade developed local recurrence.
- 15% recurrence rate for tumor size ≤ 1.5 cm
        vs.
  50% recurrence rate for tumor size 1.6–2.5 cm.
- There were no breast cancer related deaths and no patients have developed distant metastases.

Multicentricity

- Lagios series [Lagios MD, Cancer 59: 1309–1314, 1982].
  - Observed 33% incidence of multicentricity in a mammographic and pathologic study of 53 breasts removed because of DCIS.
  - Multicentricity was 3 x more frequent with DCIS > 2.6 cm.

- Schwartz [Schwartz GF, Cancer 45: 2913–2916, 1980].
  - Mammographically detected in 5 of 11 breasts removed.
  - Noted multicentricity in patients with DCIS < 1 cm in diameter.

- [Holland R, Lancet 335: 519–522, 1990]
  - 1/82 ♀ with DCIS had true multicentricity.

Radiation therapy

[Fowble B, 15th Annual International Miami Breast Cancer Conference, Febraury 26–28, 1998].

[Marks LB, Oncology 11(9): 1361–71, 1997].

[Silverstein MJ, Ductal Carcinoma in Situ. Williams and Wilkins, Baltimore, 1997].

● Collaborative study.
   [Solin LJ, J Clin Oncol 14: 754–763, 1996].
   − Nine institutions participated in the United States and Europe.
   − Analyzed outcome of 259 ♀.
   − The literature reviewing XRT and DCIS involves not only patients with mammographically detected DCIS but also DCIS associated with a palpable mass and/or bloody nipple discharge.
   − Demonstrated, at 10 years of follow-up, the actuarial breast recurrence rate was 16% after conservative surgery and XRT.
   − The 15-year actuarial breast recurrence rate was 19%.
   − The 15-year actuarial cause-specific survival was 96%.

● The studies have not clearly evaluated the effect of radiation therapy on mammographically detected DCIS.

● Currently 85% of all DCIS is detected solely as a mammographic finding.

● Collaborative group study.
   [Cancer J Sci Am 2: 158–165, 1996].
   − 110 ♀ with mammographically detected DCIS were treated with conservative surgery and XRT.
   − Median follow-up 9.3 years.
   − 14% actuarial breast recurrence rate at 10 years.
   − For patients with (−) margins at resection, the 10 year actuarial breast recurrence rate was 8%.

● There is little evidence to suggest that DCIS is inherently less radiosensitive than invasive carcinoma.

● The overall risk of developing ipsilateral <u>invasive</u> breast cancer is ∼ 5%.

- The incidence of developing a subsequent contralateral breast cancer in patients undergoing conservative surgery and XRT for DCIS is ~ 5%.

- The greatest risk factors predicting for breast recurrence in patients undergoing conservative surgery and XRT for DCIS include:

  - Residual microcalcifications on post biopsy mammograms.
    - If calcifications are left behind after resection, there is virtually a 100% risk of breast recurrence.

  - Bloody nipple discharge.

  - (+) margins at resection site.
    - Silverstein reported a 25% breast recurrence rate for margins < 1 mm, compared to a 15% for 1–9 mm margins, and 3% for margins ≥ 1 cm.
    - Collaborative group reported a 29% breast cancer recurrence rate for margins ≤ 2 mm.

  - (+) family history requires further study.

- The mean interval to a breast recurrence following conservative surgery alone ranges from 17 to 30 months.

- In patients with (−) margins, one-third were found to have residual DCIS on further surgery.

- Van Nuys Prognostic Index (VNPI).
  [Silverstein MJ, Ductal Carcinoma in Situ of the Breast, pp 491–501].
  [Silverstein MJ, Cancer 77: 2267–2274, 1996].
  - 333 ♀ were evaluated.
  - An attempt to determine which subgroup of DCIS patients would benefit from XRT after local excision.
  - This prognostic index incorporates tumor size, width of surgical excision margin, and the histologic type of DCIS into a scoring scheme.

– There are three categories for each of these factors with each assigned a score of 1–3.

– The size categories are:
  – ≤ 1.5 cm.
  – 1.6–4 cm.
  – ≥ 4.1 cm.

– The margin categories are:
  – ≥ 1 cm.
  – 1–9 mm.
  – < 1 mm.

– The pathology categories are:
  – Low grade without necrosis.
  – Low grade with necrosis.
  – High grade with or without necrosis.

– RESULTS of retrospective analysis:
  – For ♀ treated with conservative surgery and XRT the 10 year actuarial DFS was:
  – 100% for scores 3–4.
    – Lowest index score-most favorable prognosis.
    – Small tumor, wide excision margins, less aggressive pathology.
    – These ♀ did not benefit from breast XRT.

  – 77% for scores 5–7.
    – Moderate index score.
    – These ♀ did receive benefit from breast XRT.
  – 37% for scores 8–9.
    – Highest index score.
    – These ♀ derived a modest benefit from breast XRT.
    – Breast relapse rate in this group was unacceptably high with or without XRT.
    – They recommend simple mastectomy in this group.

– The VNPI needs to be further validated in large prospective Randomized clinical trials.

- Silverstein series.
  [Silverstein MJ, Eur J Cancer 28: 630–634, 1992].
  – with DCIS without microinvasion were selected.
  – Group I.
    – 98 ♀.
    – Least favorable prognostically.
    – Large lesions with (+) biopsy margins.
    – Average lesional size 3.3 cm.
    – Underwent mastectomy.
  – The most favorable, small lesions with clear margins underwent breast preservation.

  – Group II.
    – Conservative surgery + XRT.
    – Average lesional size 1.4 cm.

  – Group III.
    – Conservative surgery alone.
    – Average lesional size 1.0 cm.

  – 163 axillary dissections were done.
    – All axillary dissections were negative.
    – DCIS without microinvasion rarely metastasizes to the LNs.

  – RESULTS:
    – ♀ in Group II recurred locally at a statistically higher rate than those treated with mastectomy, in spite of the fact that ♀ in Group II had clinically more favorable lesions.
    – There was no significant difference in overall survival in any of the three groups regardless of the treatment.

	Number of patients	DFS (free from local recurrence)
Mastectomy (Group I)	98	98%
Conservative surgery + XRT (Group II)	103	84%
Conservative surgery alone (Group III)	26	67%

Rationale for radiation
[Solin LJ, J Clin Oncol 14: 754–763, 1996].
- NSABP-B06.
  [Fisher B, New Engl J Med 320: 822–28, 1989].
  [Fisher ER, J Surg Oncol 47: 139–47, 1991].
  – This is the only prospective Randomized trial comparing mastectomy to breast conservation treatment in DCIS.
  – 2072 ♀ with stage I/II invasive carcinoma.
    – A subset of these patients with DCIS was analyzed.
  – 76/2072 found to have DCIS retrospectively.
  – The majority of these ♀ presented with a palpable mass.
  – Patients randomized to:
    – Lumpectomy (L): 21/76 ♀.
    – Lumpectomy + XRT (L + XRT): 27/76 ♀.
    – Modified radical mastectomy (MRM): 28/76 ♀.
  – No patients received chemotherapy.
  – Average follow-up was 85 months.
  – Local recurrence ratio:
    – (L): 43% (9/21 ♀).
      – 56% of the recurrences were invasive.
      – 10% of these ♀ died of their disease.
    – (L + XRT): 7% (2/27 ♀).
      – 50% of the recurrences were invasive.
      – No patients in this group have died of their disease.
    – (MRM): 0% (0/28) ♀.
      – 4% of these ♀ have died of their disease.
  – Recommendations:
    – XRT may ↓ the risk of local recurrence, a large prospective Randomized clinical trial is needed.

- NSABP-B17.
  [Fisher B, New Engl J Med 328: 1581–1586, 1993].
  [Fisher ER, Cancer 75: 1310–1319, 1995].
  [Fisher B, J Clin Oncol 16: 441–452, 1998].
  – 818 patients, with localized DCIS after lumpectomy, were prospectively Randomized to receive XRT vs. observation only.
  – Recruited October 1985 to December 1990.
  – Mean time on study: 90 months (range, 67–130 months).
  – All patients are now beyond 5 years.
    – 35% of patients are beyond 8 years.

— All patients had localized DCIS, non invasive and not extensive, with reportedly histologically clear margins after removal.
— DCIS characteristics:
  — 81% were non-palpable.
    — These tumors were detected by mammography alone.
  — 50% had comedo necrosis.
— All patients had lumpectomy then Randomized to XRT (5000 rads) vs. no XRT.
— Axillary dissection done when the study began, then stopped and 2/3rds of the patients did not have axillary dissection.
— 1/3rd of the patients < 49 years old.
— 391 patients underwent lumpectomy.
— 399 patients underwent lumpectomy + radiation.
— RESULTS:
  — Subsequent ipsilateral DCIS ↓ with XRT from 13.4% (no XRT) to 8.2% (XRT). ($P = 0.007$).
  — Subsequent development of invasive breast cancer ↓ with XRT from 13.4% (no XRT) to 3.9% (XRT). ($P < 0.0001$).
  — At 8 years there was no difference in survival between the two groups.
  — The cumulative incidence of invasive contralateral breast cancer was 4.2% at 8 years of follow-up.
    — This fact speaks very strongly against performing prophylactic mastectomy of the opposite breast among DCIS patients.
    — 20 breasts would have to be removed prophylactically before finding invasive cancer in one of them.

— CONCLUSIONS:
  — Multivariate analysis showed comedo necrosis and (+) margins predicted for ipsilateral breast cancer, however, radiation after lumpectomy provided a clear benefit.
  — The size of the clustered calcification correlated with breast recurrence rates in both arms of the trial.
  — All patients benefited from radiation.

— Limitations of this study:
  — The width of the (−) margins obtained were NOT clearly defined.
  — There was no documentation of post biopsy mammograms.
  — Negative margins and a negative post biopsy mammogram are the two available ways to determine whether the DCIS was completely excised or not.

— This study provides no information with regard to the treatment of large, clinically determined DCIS.
— This information should be forthcoming in NSABP-B24.

- EORTC 10853.
  — European version of NSABP-B17.
  — 1010 ♀ with DCIS Randomized.
  Group I: Local excision alone (503 ♀).
  Group II: Local excision + XRT (507 ♀).

  — Mean age: 53 years.
  — Median diameter of lesion: 20 mm.
  — RESULTS pending publication.

- [Solin LJ, Cancer 68: 2337–2344, 1991].
  — Prospective studies of DCIS treated with lumpectomy + XRT with follow-up longer than 5 years have shown a doubling of local recurrence rates between 5–8 years of follow-up. However, this is not evaluating mammographically detected DCIS, but palpable DCIS and margins of resection were frequently unknown.

- NSABP-B24 (results submitted for publication).
  — 1804 ♀.
  — Randomized between May 1991–April 1994.
  — DCIS with extensive component.
  — All ♀ treated with lumpectomy + XRT.
  — Then randomized to tamoxifen vs. no-tamoxifen.
  — There is a reported 5% benefit to the tamoxifen arm.

LCIS (Lobular Carcinoma *In Situ*)
[Zurrida S, Ann Surg Oncol 3(1):57–61 1996].
[Horiguchi J, Oncology 51: 47–51, 1994].

- It is usually an incidental finding in premenopausal ♀ 35–55 years old with fibrocystic changes.

- Less common in African Americans.

- Generally involves multiple lobules (multifocal or diffuse).

- It is not cancer.

- Never produces a mass; it is a microscopic entity only.

- A negative aspirate certainly does not exclude LCIS.

- No clinical or mammographic presentation.

- Frozen section is unreliable because there is no grossly visible lesion to direct the sampling.

- Proven to be diploid in most cases.

- Typically is ER(+), does not show c-erbB-2 expression and has a very low proliferative rate.

- Risk of subsequent development of invasive cancer in either breast is 1–1.5% per year.
  - Risk of 20–30% in lifetime, equally divided among breasts.

- The mean interval for the development of an invasive carcinoma, either ipsilateral or contralateral, is approximately 15–20 years.

- [Bodian CA, Cancer 78: 1024–1034, 1996].
  - 236 ♀ with lobular neoplasia were studied.
  - Median follow-up of 18 years.
  - Conclusion:
    - ~ 1/3rd of the ♀ would probably develop carcinoma with longterm follow-up, which is 5.4 × the rate in the general population.
    - The relative risk decreased with increasing age at diagnosis.
  - The risks for subsequent development of carcinoma remain high for at least 20 years and ↑ substantially if there was a second biopsy (+) for lobular neoplasia.

- ♀ with LCIS and with the highest relative risk of developing invasive cancer are:
  - ♀ years of age.
  - ♀ s/p two breast biopsies with the second biopsy (+) for LCIS.

- Only 1/2 of the subsequent carcinomas that will develop will be lobular carcinomas, the other half will be ductal carcinomas.

Treatment

- Observation vs. chemoprevention trials.
  - Such as the Breast Cancer Prevention Trial (BCPT).
    - NSABP-P1 tamoxifen chemoprevention trial.
    - Closed September 1997.
  - For more details, refer to the Chemoprevention section on page 165.

- No role for chemotherapy or radiation.

- Prophylactic bilateral simple mastectomies usually with immediate reconstruction is the surgical procedure of choice if the patient has decided to have surgery.

INVASIVE CANCER

SURGICAL TREATMENT

STAGE I/II OPERABLE BREAST CANCER
[Harris JR, New Engl J Med 327(6): 390–398, 1992].

Lumpectomy

- Lumpectomy (tumorectomy).
  - 1 cm margin of normal tissue removed en bloc.

- The more peripheral the carcinoma and the larger the breast, the easier the conservation and the less deformity.

Quadrantectomy

- Quadrantectomy (segmentectomy).
  - 3 cm margin of normal tissue removed en bloc with a portion of overlying skin and the underlying muscular fascia.
  - Muscles are not removed.
  - Designed to address the segmental growth pattern of breast cancer.

Mastectomy

- Radical mastectomy (RM) = removal of the breast + pectoralis major and minor muscles.

- Modified radical mastectomy (MRM) = removal of the breast, but spares pectoralis major and the lateral pectoral nerve ± pectoralis minor muscle.
  - Modified radical mastectomy = radical mastectomy (if pectoralis major muscle is not involved) in terms of survival.

- Distant metastases are a relative contraindication for mastectomy.

- Complications of mastectomy:
  - Wound infection.
    - Cellulitis.
    - Abscess formation.

— Necrosis of skin flaps.
  — Rare.
— Seroma formation.
  [Burak WE, J Surg Oncol 64: 27–31, 1997].
  — Occurs in ~ 100% of patients.
— Changes in chest wall sensation.
— Phantom breast syndrome.
  — Can last for years.
— Post-surgical pain syndrome.
— Lymphedema.

Mastectomy vs. breast-conserving therapy

● [Keynes G, Br Med J 2: 643–647, 1937].
  — Dr Geoffrey Keynes, a surgeon at St. Barthomew's Hospital in London, began treating operative breast cancer patients conservatively in 1924.

● Local excision with radiotherapy produces equivalent results, in terms of survival, when compared to mastectomy.
  — Proven by seven Randomized trials.
— [NCI Consensus Conference, J Am Med Assoc 265: 391–395, 1991].
  — CONCLUSION: Breast conserving treatment is an appropriate primary therapy for the majority of ♀ with stage I/II breast cancer.

● Lumpectomy with level I and II axillary LN dissection + XRT = total mastectomy + axillary LN dissection:
  If tumor T < 4 cm.
  And clear margins.

● Currently there is no consensus regarding the optimal extent of surgery required (Lumpectomy vs. Quadrantectomy) before irradiation.
  — The approach is influenced by the size of the area to be resected and relative to the size of the patient's breast.

● [Early Breast Cancer Trialists Collaborative Group (EBCTCG), New Engl J Med 333: 1444–1455, 1995].
  — Overview (meta-analyses) of Randomized trials of local therapies for early breast cancer looks at effects on mortality and local recurrence.
  — Addition of XRT to surgery decreased local recurrence rate, but overall survival was the same in 10 years.

Breast conserving therapy: Randomized trials			
Institution	Years	No. of patients M = mastectomy L = lumpectomy XRT = radiation therapy	Overall survival %
Milan [1]	1973– 1980	349 (M) 352 (XRT)	65 (18 years) 65
NSABP-B06 [2]	1976– 1984	590 (M) 629 (L+XRT)	60 (12 years) 62
Danish BCG [3]	1983– 1987	429 (M) 430 (XRT)	82 (6 years) 79
Gustav-Roussy [4]	1972– 1979	91 (M) 88 (XRT)	65 (15 years) 73
NCI [5,6]	1980– 1986	116 (M) 121 (XRT)	75 (10 years) 77
EORTC [7]	1980– 1986	426 (M) 456 (XRT)	63 (8 years) 58
Guy's Hospital [8]	1981– 1986	185 (M) 214 (XRT)	Equal (54 months)

[1] [Veronesi U, Eur J Cancer 31A: 1574–1579, 1995].
[2] [Fisher B, New Engl J Med 333: 1456–1461, 1995].
[3] [Blichert-Toft MJ, Natl Cancer Inst Monographs 11: 19–25, 1992].
[4] [Arriagada R, J Clin Oncol 14: 1558–1564, 1996].
[5] [Lichter AS, J Clin Oncol 10: 976–983, 1992].
[6] [Jacobson JA, New Engl J Med 332: 907–911, 1995].
[7] [vanDongen JA, J Natl Cancer Inst Monographs 11: 15–18, 1992].
[8] [Chaudry MA, Breast Cancer Res Treat 14: 140, 1989].

- NSABP-B06
  [Fisher B, New Engl J Med 320: 822–828, 1989].
  [Fisher B, New Engl J Med 333: 1456–1461, 1995].
  – First US trial to prove that Lumpectomy + axillary node dissection + XRT [L + A + XRT] = MRM.
  – Total of 2163 patients.
  – All patients had (–) margins after lumpectomy or underwent mastectomy.

— ~ 1200 patients with tumor size ≤ 4 cm and LN(−).
— Follow-up at 12 years.

	Local recurrence (%)		Survival %
	LN(+)	LN(−)	
MRM			60
Lumpectomy+ axillary dissection	41 (+chemotherapy)	32	58
Lumpectomy + axillary dissection+ radiotherapy	5 (+chemotherapy)	12	62

— All LN(+) patients received chemotherapy (Melphalan and 5FU).
— XRT = 50 Gy over 5 weeks, no boost.
— Local recurrence.
  — 1%/year with [L + XRT].
  — 4–5%/year with lumpectomy without XRT.
— In patients who received lumpectomy alone, with clear margins, there was a local recurrence rate of 27% after 5 years vs. 9% with [L + A + XRT].
— Disease free survival is equal for MRM and [L + A + XRT].
— CONCLUSION:
  — At 12 years, data continues to indicate that [L + A + XRT] + adjuvant chemotherapy in LN(+) ♀ is appropriate therapy for stage I/II breast cancer provided margins of resected specimens are free of tumor.

• Milan I
  [Veronesi U, Eur J Cancer 31A(10): 1574–1579, 1995].
  [Veronesi U, Eur J Cancer 26: 668–670, 1990].
  — Randomized trial 1973–1980.
  — 701 ♀ with stage I/II breast cancer < 70 years old.
  — 349 patients received Halsted mastectomy (24.6% (+)LN).
  — 352 patients received UART (quadrantectomy + axillary dissection + XRT to the breast) (27% (+)LN).
  — XRT = 50 Gy with 10 Gy boost.

- After 1976 all patients with (+)LN received CMF × 12 months.
- In 1981 early results showed clear evidence of similar survival curves with the two procedures.
- In 1995 final evaluation of the 18-year survival data showed identical results for the two procedures. (Overall survival 65% vs. 65%, respectively).
- Subdivisions of patients by size of tumor, site and age, did not reveal any difference between the treatments.
- CONCLUSION:
  - No role for total mastectomy in patients with small size carcinomas.

- **Milan II**
  [Veronesi U, Eur J Cancer 31A(10): 1574–1579, 1995].
  [Veronesi U, Eur J Cancer 26(6): 671–673, 1990].
  - Randomized trial 1985–1987.
  - Quadrantectomy + total axillary dissection and radiotherapy (QUART) vs. tumorectomy (lumpectomy) + total axillary dissection followed by XRT (TART).
  - External radiation was started 4–6 weeks after surgery.
  - A dose of 60 Gy given to both groups of patients.
  - Nodal sites were never irradiated.
  - 705 patients were evaluable with stage I/II breast cancer (up to 2.5 cm size primary tumors).
    - 360 were treated with QUART.
    - 345 treated with TART.
  - Last review (1994) shows 15 local recurrences in the QUART group and 39 in the TART group.
    - Patients with positive margins + XRT → 20% local recurrence.
    - Majority of these patients had EIC.
  - The incidence of distant metastases (36 patients vs. 35 patients) and survival is identical in the two groups.
  - CONCLUSIONS:
    - Conservative surgery should include generous negative margins and post-op XRT.
    - The patient should decide whether a higher rate of local recurrence is an acceptable price for better cosmetic result.

- **Milan III**
  [Veronesi U, Eur J Cancer 31A(10): 1574–1579, 1995].
  [Veronesi U, New Engl J Med 328: 1587–1591, 1993].

- Randomized trial 1987–1988 to evaluate efficacy of quadrantectomy with or without post-op XRT (50 Gy to breast with 10 Gy boost to tumor bed).
- 579 patients:
  - 294 ♀ treated with quadrantectomy + axillary dissection and XRT.
  - 273 ♀ treated with quadrantectomy + axillary dissection and no XRT.
- Median follow-up 39 months.
- Incidence of local recurrence was 8.8% (24/273 patients) among patients treated with quadrantectomy <u>without</u> XRT compared with 0.3% (1/294 patients) among patients treated <u>with</u> XRT. ($P =$ 0.001).
- Increased incidence of local recurrence in the group that did not receive XRT was associated with young age and the presence of EIC.
  - Recurrence rate was 17.5% in patients < 45 years old and 3.8% in patients > 55 years old.
  - Patients with EIC had local recurrence of 16.7 vs. 7.4% in patients who did not.
- The 4-year overall survival was similar in the 2 groups.
- CONCLUSION:
  - XRT after quadrantectomy reduces the risk of local recurrence.

- CONCLUSIONS of Milan II/III studies:
  [Veronesi U, World J Surg 18: 70–75, 1994] (Figs. 6–8).
  - ↑ volume of resection will ↓ local recurrence, but ↓ cosmetic results.
  - XRT very effective.
  - XRT markedly decreases risk of local recurrence even if margins are negative because of the rate of false (−) margins.
  - False negative results among patients with clear margins are seen because of multifocal cancer lesions beyond the margin.
  - 40% false (−) rate found among patients with (−) margins.
  - The finding of clear margins should not abolish additional treatments like XRT.
  - (+) margins → 2 × risk of local recurrence.
  - Extending resection to 3 cm decreases (+) margins by 2/3rds.
  - In patients with EIC → re-excision with a clear margin is necessary prior to commencing XRT.

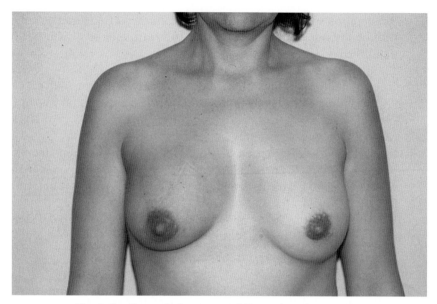

Fig. 6. Excellent esthetic outcome of Veronesi quadrantectomy.

● In most (conservative surgery + XRT) studies the local recurrence rate is
  ～1% per year.

● Risks for local recurrence after (conservative surgery + XRT)
  — Age
    — < 35 years old—↑ risk.
  — Extent of surgery.
    — Clean margins, ↓ risk.
  — Chemotherapy.
    — Improves local control, synergistic with XRT.
    — ↓ risk.

● Contraindications to lumpectomy/XRT
  [Winchester DP, CA Cancer J Clin 42: 134–162, 1992].
  — Options must be discussed with the patient.
    — When asked, 80% of the patients will choose lumpectomy + XRT
    over mastectomy.

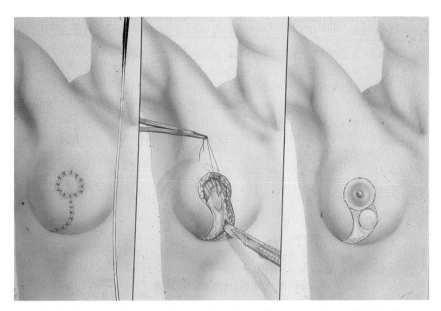

Fig. 7. Three principal steps in central quadrantectomy according to Galimberti.

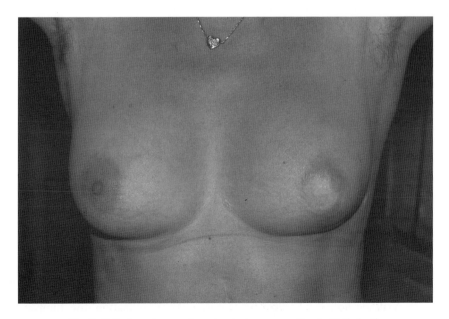

Fig. 8. Esthetic outcome of quadrantectomy according to Galimberti.

— Absolute contraindications:

  — 1st, 2nd or 3rd trimester pregnancy.
    — Patient must deliver prior to XRT.
  — Prior radiation to the breast.
  — Two or more gross malignancies in separate quadrants of the same breast.
  — Extensive diffuse mammographic areas suspicious for malignancy (calcifications).

— Relative contraindications:

  — Very large and very small breasts.
    — Tumor/breast ratio.
    — Tumor > 4–5 cm.
  — Subareolar (central) tumor.
    — Unless it can be completely excised.

  [Galimberti V, Eur J Cancer 29a(8): 1093–1096, 1993].
    — Centrally located small tumors are no longer an absolute indication for mastectomy.
    — A central quadrantectomy has been described among 37 ♀ achieving the same radicality as in other quadrants and good cosmetic results with plastic surgery remodelling.

  — Extensive intraductal component.
    — With (+) margins after repeated resections.
    — With (−) excission margins it is not a contraindication.

  — Collagen vascular disorder.
    — There are six case reports in the literature of subsequent development of acute severe fibrosis to the breast after XRT.
      — Scleroderma.
      — Lupus.
      — Rheumatoid arthritis (controversial).
  — Ataxia-telangiectasia patients and carriers of the gene.

— Axillary nodal involvement is not a contraindication for lumpectomy + XRT.

— Breast cancer arising in ♀ previously treated with irradiation above the diaphragm for lymphoma is not a contraindication for lumpectomy + XRT. [Karasek K, Am J Clin Oncol 19: 451–454, 1996].

— ♀ with synchronous or metachronous bilateral breast cancers are also eligible for breast conserving therapy. [Gollamudi SV, Cancer 79: 1362–1369, 1997].

● Role of a radiation boost.
  [Romestaing P, J Clin Oncol 15: 963–968, 1997].
  — 1024 ♀ with breast cancer tumor ≤ 3 cm in diameter.
  — Treated between 1986–1992.
  — Underwent local excision, axillary dissection and conventional 50 Gy irradiation, given in 20 fractions over 5 weeks to the whole breast.
  — Then Randomized to: no further treatment vs. a 10 Gy boost by electrons to the tumor bed.
  — At 5 years: 10/521 patients that had received the boost had a local recurrence. (3.6%)
            vs. 20/503 patients (4.5%) who had not received the boost.
    ($P = 0.044$).
  — The boost group had a higher rate of grade 1 and 2 telangiectasia (12.4% vs. 5.9%).
  — CONCLUSION:
    — A 10 Gy boost to the tumor bed, after 50 Gy to the whole breast, following breast conserving surgery, significantly ↓ risk of early local recurrence, with no serious deterioration in the cosmetic outcome.

● Poor cosmetic outcome.
  — Large resections in small breast.
  — Whole breast radiation > 50 Gy.
  — Daily radiation dose > 2 Gy/day.
  — Overlapping fields.

● Complications of radiation therapy.
  — The risk of complications after XRT is much higher in ♀ who receive chemotherapy.

— Prolonged breast edema.

— Ipsilateral arm lymphedema.
  — Chronic infections.

— Paresthesias.
  — Brachial plexopathy.

— ↓ arm mobility.

— Soft tissue necrosis, fibrosis.

— Rib fractures.

— Angiosarcoma.
  [Cafiero F, Cancer 77: 2496–2502, 1996].
  [Wijnmaalen A', Int J Radiat Oncol Biol Phys, 26: 135–139, 1993].
  — Very rare since radiation techniques have changed.
  — But can occur after XRT.
  — A confounding factor is chronic lymphedema.
  — Cumulative risk of sarcoma is < 1% in 30 years.

— Ipsilateral lung cancer.
  [Neugut AI, Cancer 71: 3054–3057, 1993].
  — Uncommon.
  — ↑ in smokers.

— Esophageal cancer.
  [Ahsan H, Ann Intern Med 128: 114–117, 1998].
  — ↑ risk of esophageal cancer, 10 or more years after XRT is
    completed.
  — This study is based on small numbers and did not have available
    information on the dose of XRT given or other factors such as
    smoking history, alcohol intake or whether or not the patient had
    received chemotherapy.
  — This study did not address the issue of technical improvements in
    XRT over the past 20 years.
  — Internal mammary nodes are less likely to be routinely irradiated
    today and this is the field which includes the esophagus.
  — The findings of this study apply more to women who received
    XRT in the past and are now being seen in follow-up.

— Coronary artery disease.
  — Believed to be a lesser problem now, with the use of tangential beams and modern techniques.

— Symptomatic pneumonitis.
  — ↑ risk when the direct internal mammary field is involved.
  — Typically presents 3–12 months after XRT, with dry cough, shortness of breath and low grade fever.

- Radiation after lumpectomy.
  — 5–7 weeks in duration.

- Lumpectomy with or without XRT?
[Clark RM, J Natl Cancer Inst 88: 1659–1664, 1996].
[Forrest AP, Lancet 348: 708–713, 1996].
  — Among the Randomized trials comparing lumpectomy with or without XRT, to date, there has <u>not</u> been a patient subgroups identified where the XRT can be 'safely' omitted.
  — Whether or not a certain group of ♀ with breast cancer can be safely spared XRT after lumpectomy remains to be determined.
  — Two ongoing trials in the U.S. test whether tamoxifen can be substituted for XRT in order to ↓ local recurrences in ♀ with low-risk breast cancer.
    — NSABP-B21.
    — CALGB 9343.
      — Focusses on older ♀.

- Quadrantectomy with or without XRT?
  — EORTC 10932.
    —Ongoing Randomized trial comparing quadrantectomy with and without XRT.
    —♀ > 50 years of age, LN(−), with tumors that have a grade I histology and are < 2 cm in size, without evidence of vascular invasion or extensive DCIS, qualify.

- Extensive intraductal component (EIC).

  — Definition.
    — > 25% of tumor volume is DCIS <u>and</u> DCIS extends beyond borders of <u>invasive</u> disease.
    —DCIS with microinvasion.

- Larger resection required.

- Re-excision, then XRT if clear margins obtained.

- If not clear → consider mastectomy.

- XRT is less able to eradicate large areas of DCIS or invasive ductal carcinoma, at cosmetically acceptable doses.

- Timing of breast surgery.
  [Davidson NE, Cancer Treat Rev 19: 105–112, 1993].
  - Optimal timing of resection in relation to the menstrual cycle is controversial and in premenopausal ♀ is an issue that merits further evaluation in a prospective Randomized trial [McGuire WL, Annals of Int Med 115: 401–403, 1992].
  - Some studies have shown resections performed during perimenstrual phase (days 0–6, 21–36 from the start of last period) were associated with significantly greater recurrence rate than resections performed during periovulatory phase (days 7–20).
  - This finding has not been observed in other large studies.

  [Veronesi U, 15th International Miami Breast Cancer Conference, February 26–28, 1998].
  - Other studies have shown ♀ having surgery during the first 14 days of the cycle (follicular phase) seem to have a higher recurrence rate than those treated during the second phase of the cycle (luteal phase).
  - In 1994 at the NCI-Milan, 1175 premenopausal ♀ were surgically treated for breast cancer.
  - A retrospective review has been conducted.
  - In this study:
    - Premenopausal ♀ with breast cancer and (+)LNs operated on during the luteal phase had a significantly better prognosis than ♀ operated on during the follicular phase.
    - This retrospective review could have been affected by many variables, so a large prospective trial has been initiated.
    - Premenopausal ♀ younger than 48 years old with breast cancer < 5 cm in diameter are being accepted for this study.
    - The patients are self-randomized to one of two groups.
      - Follicular phase.
      - Luteal phase.
    - ~ 800 ♀ are needed to complete this study; 390 ♀ have been entered to-date.

POST-MASTECTOMY RADIOTHERAPY

[Lichter AS, Diseases of the Breast Updates 1(4): 1–10, 1997].
[Overgaard M, New Engl J Med 337: 949–955, 1997].
[Ragaz J, New Engl J Med 337: 956–962, 1997].
[Fowble B, Oncology 11: 213–239, 1997].
[Ragaz J, Proc Am Soc Clin Oncol 6: 121(A150), 1987].
[Arriagada R, J Clin Oncol 13: 2869–2878, 1995].

- The most common sites of loco-regional failure after mastectomy are the chest wall, the supraclavicular LNs, and the axilla (if initial surgery was limited).
  − 40% of chest wall recurrences occur in mastectomy scar.

- The loco-regional failure rate following mastectomy is often very high (10–30%), especially in patients with multiple (+)LNs.

- [Valagussa P, Cancer 41: 1170–1178, 1978].
  − Tumor size has strongly been correlated with loco-regional recurrence in LN(+) patients.

- Loco-regional recurrences can be difficult to control.
  − With an average control rate of ∼ 50%.
  − Thus it is preferable to prevent them.

- Some of the controversy in this topic arises from the fact that there has been a wide variability in radiation techniques and radiation doses used (at times suboptimal) in the 9 post-mastectomy Randomized trials done prior to the two reported trials in the New England Journal of Medicine in 1997.
  − One finding has remained constant in all of these pre-1997 trials.
    − ↓ in local chest wall recurrence following XRT.
  − Some but not all of the trials found an ↑ DFS.
  − None of these pre-1997 Randomized trials produced a significant ↑ OS.

- 1987 Meta-analysis.
  [Cuzick J, Cancer Treat Rep 71: 15–25, 1987].
  − In 1987 an updated meta-analysis was published.
    − It confirmed that there was no ↑ survival in patients receiving post-mastectomy radiation with 10 years of follow-up.

- After 10 years the survival curves began to diverge with the XRT patients actually doing worse.

- Cause-specific mortalities.
  [Cuzick J, J Clin Oncol 12: 447–453, 1994].
  - 1994, the cause-specific mortalities of the previous 1987 meta-analyses were reported along with that of other trials.
    - An excess in late cardiac deaths explained the detrimental effects of XRT.
    - In this newer report the difference in OS was no longer statistically significant.
    - In more recent trials, employing modern XRT techniques, they noted ↓ breast cancer deaths and ↓ in excess cardiac mortality.

- Early Breast Cancer Trialists Collaborative Group (1995 Meta-analysis).

- [EBCTCG, New Engl J Med 333: 1444–1455, 1995].
  - The most recent meta-analysis.
  - Showed a non-significant reduction of 2.6% in the odds of death for patients receiving XRT, compared with those who did not.

- [Fowble B, Oncology 10: 1–19, 1996].
  [EBCTCG, New Engl J Med 333: 1444–1455, 1995].
  - Local radiation therapy after mastectomy markedly reduces the risk of loco-regional failure to ~ 5–10%.
  - Disease-free survival is improved in pre- and postmenopausal ♀.

- The Danish Breast Cancer Cooperative Group Trial.
  [Overgaard M, New Engl J Med 337: 949–955, 1997].
  - 1708 premenopausal ♀ randomized.
  - 92% ♀ with LN(+).
  - All ♀ were treated with MRM and axillary LN sampling.
  - All ♀ were treated with CMF chemotherapy.
  - 852 ♀ randomized to receive XRT:
    - XRT included chest wall, supraclavicular LNs, and internal mammary nodes.
  - 856 ♀ randomized to no XRT.

  - Follow-up 10 years.

  - Loco-regional recurrence ↓ in the XRT arm.
    - 32 vs. 9%.

— DFS significant ↑ for the XRT arm.
— 48 vs. 34%; $P < 0.0001$.

— OS significantly ↑ for the XRT arm.
— 54 vs. 45%; $P < 0.001$.

— CONCLUSION:
— The addition of post-mastectomy radiation therapy to adjuvant chemotherapy improved overall survival by ∼ 10% at 10 years in premenopausal ♀ with positive nodes detected with axillary sampling or tumors > 5 cm.
— In all LN(+) patients this survival benefit was similar irrespective of the number of positive LNs.
— Following mastectomy, there appeared to be a subset of (+) LN patients with microscopic residual cancer in the unresected nodes in the upper axilla, supraclavicular fossa, internal mammary nodes or chest wall without distant metastatic spread. (See 1997 New England Journal citations in table below).

— Limitations of the study:
— Few axillary LNs were removed.
— On average 7 LNs per patient.
— Likely that many ♀ had disease left in the axilla or the number of (+)LNs were underestimated.

— Small number of LNs removed made it almost impossible to determine which specific group of LN(+) ♀ would derive benefit from XRT.

● British Columbia Trial.
[Ragaz J, New Engl J Med 337: 956–962, 1997].
— 318 premenopausal ♀ with LN(+) breast cancer.
— All ♀ underwent MRM + axillary LN dissection.
— Median number of axillary LNs removed was 11.
— Then randomized:
— Group I—CMF + XRT
       vs.
— Group II-CMF alone.
— The XRT included chest wall, regional LNs and internal mammary nodes.

- Median follow-up 12.5 years.
- The results are identical to those of the Danish Trial.
- DFS at 15 years ↑ from 33 to 50% by adding XRT. ($P = 0.007$).
- OS at 15 years ↑ from 46 to 54% by adding XRT. ($P = 0.07$).
- Cause-specific survival at 15 years ↑ from 47 to 57% by adding XRT ($P = 0.05$).
- The beneficial effects of XRT were seen in ♀ with 1–3 (+)LNs as well as in those ♀ with ≥ 4(+) LNs.

Post-mastectomy radiation therapy: Four large selected Randomized trials in premenopausal and postmenopausal ♀					
Study	Number of patients	Systemic therapy	Surgery	Disease free survival	Overall survival
Stockholm (16 years) [1]	970	None	MRM	(+)XRT → 39 (−)XRT → 22 (P<0.01)	(+)XRT → 42 (−)XRT → 33 (P<0.21)
Danish (DBCG # 82) (10 years) [2] (only pre-meno ♀)	1708	CMF i.v. (9 mos)	MRM	(+)XRT → 48 (−)XRT → 34 (P<0.001)	(+)XRT → 54 (−)XRT → 45 (P<0.001)
Oslo (15 years) [3]	1115	None	RM	(+)XRT → 33 (−)XRT → 32	Equivalent
British Columbia (15 years) [4], (only pre-meno ♀)	318	CMF (12 mos)	MRM	(+)XRT → 50 (−)XRT → 33 (P<0.007)	(+)XRT → 54 (−)XRT → 46 (P<0.07)

[1] [Rutqvist LE, Radiother Oncol 26: 104–110, 1993].
[2] [Overgaard M, New Engl J Med 337: 949–955, 1997].
[3] [Host H, Int J Radiat Oncol Biol Phys 12: 727–732, 1986].
[4] [Ragaz J, New Engl J Med 337: 956–962, 1997].

- CONCLUSION:
  - The risk of loco-regional recurrence, following mastectomy, seems to be the same with or without adjuvant chemotherapy or endocrine therapy.
    - Premenopausal ♀ with (+) axillary LNs and T_3 tumors are especially at high risk.

— The use of post-mastectomy XRT reduces loco-regional failure, improves disease-free survival and overall survival.

- Recommendations for post-mastectomy XRT:
  - 50 Gy over 5 weeks, to the chest wall and supraclavicular fossa.
  - An additional 10 Gy boost to the scar in ♀ with stage III disease or (+) chest wall surgical margins can be considered, but is not standard.
    - All premenopausal ♀ with ≥ 4 (+)LNs.
    - Consideration given to premenopausal ♀ with 1–3 (+)LNs, with inadequate axillary dissection.
    - ♀ with locally advanced disease (stage III disease).
    - ♀ with (+) chest wall surgical margins.
    - It is not yet clear what to do with postmenopausal ♀ with (+) LNs.
  - Whether internal mammary nodes should be irradiated is highly controversial.

  - Both the Danish Study and the British Columbia Study included the mammary nodes in the field of radiation, however the survival benefit cannot be specifically attributed to internal mammary node treatment.

  - Some authors advocate including in the radiotherapy field the internal mammary LNs that are within the first three intercostal spaces, allowing the radiation field to end above the level of the majority of the heart, thus sparing future cardiac morbidity.

  - EORTC 22922.
    - Randomized ongoing study to specifically determine whether internal mammary nodes should be included in the radiotherapy field.

AXILLARY LYMPH NODE DISSECTION
[Kilkenny JW, Current Opinion in Oncology 9(6): 520–526, 1997].
[Hicken NF, Surg Gynecol Obstet 64: 593–603, 1937].

- It was determined via ductograms that the breast ductal system drains into the axilla 95% of the time.

- The role of axillary LN dissection is in evolution.
  – It may be avoidable in certain breast cancer patients.
  [Greco M, Anticancer Research 16: 3913–3918, 1996].

- Axillary LN dissection is mandatory when palpable axillary LNs are present, to prevent the local complications of uncontrolled tumor growth.

[Morrow M. Semin Surg Oncol 12: 321–327, 1996].
- The incidence of axillary LN metastases is related to tumor size, and lymphatic or vascular invasion.
  – (+)LN in 15–25% of ♀ with tumors ≤ 1 cm in diameter.
  – (+)LN in 3–28% of ♀ with tumors ≤ 0.5 cm in diameter.

- There are three groups recognized to-date with a very low risk for axillary metastases.
  – DCIS.
  – Microinvasive cancer.
  – Pure tubular carcinoma < 1 cm in diameter.

DCIS
[Winchester DP, Ann Surg Oncol 2: 207–213, 1995].

- Axillary node dissection is <u>not</u> indicated for patients with microscopic DCIS, since the incidence of metastases in LNs is close to 0.
  – Silverstein [Silverstein MJ, Cancer 59: 1819–1824, 1987].
    – 100 patients with axillary LN dissection.
      – 41% palpable DCIS → 0 (+)LN.
  – Wobbes [Wobbes T, Br J Surg 76: 185–186, 1989].
    – 28 patients with axillary node dissection.
      – Non-palpable DCIS → 0 (+)LN.
  – Lagios [Lagios, Cancer 50: 1309–1314, 1982].
    – 53 patients with axillary node dissection.
      – 54% palpable DCIS → 1.8% (+)LN.

- Axillary dissection may have a role in patients with palpable or radiologically extensive DCIS, since the incidence of axillary LN involvement varies from 0–21%.
  [Haagensen, Disease of the Breast, WB Saunders Co. 1986, p 782].
  - ♀ with radiologically extensive DCIS (≥ 5 cm) usually have invasive breast cancer; if LN's are (+) they have or have had invasive breast cancer.

Invasive carcinoma
- T_1a lesions.

  - Axillary LN dissection.
  - Controversial, but still the standard of care.
  - (+)LN in 3–11% of patients.

  - [Friedman NS, Proc Am Soc Clin Oncol 13: 83 (A134), 1994].
    - Dr Silverstein proposed to eliminate axillary LN dissection in all T_1a lesions and T_1b non-palpable lesions.

  - [Chontos AJ, J Am Coll Surg 184: 493–498, 1997].
    - Single institution study.
    - 256 T_1a lesions reviewed.
    - Incidence of (+) axillary LNs was 3.9%.

  - [White RE, J Am Coll Surg 183: 575–582, 1996].
    - State registry of 1126 ♀ with breast cancers < 1 cm in diameter.
    - (+)LN in 10% of T_1a tumors.
    - (+)LN in 19% of T_1b tumors.
    - LN status significantly influenced disease-free survival among these patients.

NSABP B04
[Fisher B, New Engl J Med 312(11): 674–681, 1985].

- Clinically LN(−) patients randomized to three arms:
  - Group I: mastectomy + LN dissection.
  - Group II: mastectomy + XRT to axilla.
  - Group III: mastectomy alone.
- Group III (mastectomy alone).
  - If < 5 LNs removed → 12% axillary recurrence rate.
  - If > 5 LNs removed → 0% axillary recurrence rate.

	Group I (%)	Group II (%)	Group III (%)
10 year overall survival	58	59	54
15 year overall survival	45	46	41

- Because of the 10-year results, axillary dissections have been done for prognostic information.

- In ~ 5% of patients, LN dissection may be therapeutic.
  - This was evident with the 15 year OS results of NSABP-B04.

  - In the Guy's Hospital Trial [Hayward J, Arch Surg 122: 1244–1247, 1987].
    - Patients with poorly irradiated axillas had an ↑ rate of metastases and a worse overall survival.

- [Fisher B, Surg Gynecol and Obstet 129: 705–716, 1969].
  - Patients with lateral tumors are more likely to have positive axillary lymph nodes when compared to patients with medial tumors.

Complications of axillary LN dissection
  - Injury or thrombosis of axillary vein (rare).
  - Injury to the motor nerves of the axilla.
  - Seroma formation.
  - Shoulder dysfunction.
  - Loss of sensation in the distribution of the intercostobrachial nerve.

  - Lymphedema of the breast and of the arm.
    [Morrow M. Semin Surg Oncol 12: 321–327, 1996].
    - Incidence ranges between 10–20% in modern surgical series.
    - Operated ♀ remain at risk the rest of their lives.

Lymphatic mapping

- Sentinel node biopsy.
  [Turner RR, Ann Surg 226: 271–278, 1997].
  [Albertini JJ, J Am Med Assoc 276: 1818–1822, 1996].
  [Statman R, Adv Surg 30: 209–221, 1996].
  [Anon, Oncology 9(8): 722, 1995].
  [Giuliano AE, Ann Surg 220: 391–398, 1994].

— The sentinel node is the lymph node most likely to harbor metastases in the axilla if the tumor has spread.

— Lymphatic mapping techniques may avoid axillary dissections in the future by identifying the sentinel lymph node, as is done in patients with melanoma.

— Based on the theory that:
  — Lymph drainage including metastases will lead to the sentinel lymph node.
  — Examination and dissection of the sentinel lymph node will provide sufficient information as to the diagnosis and stage of disease in order to avoid total axillary lymph node dissection, along with the morbidity to the patient and the cost.

  — The two current techniques include mapping with either an isosulfan blue dye or a radiolabeled gamma probe or both.

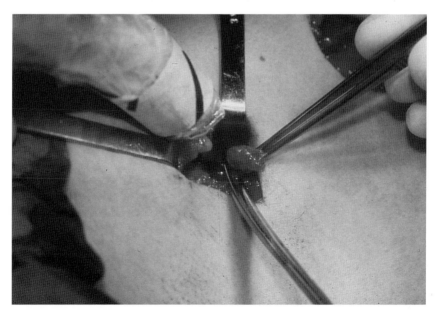

Fig. 9. Intraoperative localisation of sentinel node using gamma ray-detecting probe.

- A learning curve for this technique is clearly present.
  - With blue dye alone the sentinel LN was identified:
    - 59% of the first 87 procedures.
    - 78% of the last 50 procedures.
  - Currently has a sensitivity of 88% and a specificity of 100%.

- Ongoing studies on both sides of the Atlantic are trying to determine whether removal of one lymph node from the axilla, 'the sentinel node', is sufficient for staging.

- The Sentinel node would be the one that receives the majority of the lymphatic drainage from the tumor bed in the breast.

- If pathological evaluation of the sentinel node proves to be efficacious, level I/II axillary dissections will become obsolete but for now, axillary lymph node dissection provides valuable information and remains the standard.

- [Veronesi U, Lancet 349: 1864–1867, 1997].
  - 163 consecutive ♀ with operable breast cancer were entered into this study.
  - The cancer was newly diagnosed, non-metastatic, invasive, and operable.
  - Previous to their axillary LN dissection, the ♀ had a tracer subdermally injected.
  - A radiolabelled gamma probe was used to identify the sentinel node (Fig. 9).
  - The sentinel node was removed prior to the axillary LN dissection.
  - Sentinel node analysis was possible in 160 (98%) of the 163 ♀.

  - The sentinel node accurately predicted axillary LN status:
    - In 156 (97.5%) of the 160 ♀.
      - There were 4 ♀ identified with 'skip' metastases in which the sentinel LN was (−) but there were other (+) axillary LNs.
    - In 45 (100%) of the ♀ with tumors < 1.5 cm in diameter.
    - In 32 (38%) of the 85 ♀ with metastatic axillary LN, the only (+)LN was the sentinel node.

- Technical caveats of sentinel LN biopsy.
  [Statmen R, Adv Surg 30: 209–221, 1996].

[Giuliano AE, 15th International Miami Breast Cancer Meeting, February 26–28, 1998].

— Avoid large biopsy cavities.

— Patients with large tumors are not good candidates for sentinel LN dissection.

— Time the axillary incision and dissection correctly.
   — The transit time from an upper-outer-quadrant carcinoma to the sentinel node is shorter than the transit time from a lower-inner-quadrant carcinoma.
   — 3–7 min should be timed by the clock.

— Identify the blue-impregnated lymphatic channel before attempting to identify the sentinel node.
   — The sentinel node may be level II instead of level I.

— Obtain pre-operative lymphoscintigrams for patients with medial hemisphere lesions.
   — The lesion may drain only into the internal mammary nodes, hence an axillary sentinel LN dissection should not be attempted.
   — ∼ 5–10% of LN(−) ♀ have (+) internal mammary LNs, most originating from inner quadrant tumors.

— Inject the tumor or cavity prior to incising the breast.
   — It is essential that the lymphatic system remains closed.

[Rosen PP, Ann Surg 197: 276–283, 1983].
[Veronesi U, Cancer 59: 682–687, 1987].

— Lymphatic mapping does not address the issue of 'skip' metastases.

— In the above mentioned studies, the incidence of isolated metastases to Level III axillary LNs with (−) Level I–II axillary LNs was very low.
   — Ranging from 0.2–0.4%.

— In the above mentioned studies, the incidence of isolated metastases to Level II axillary LNs with (−) Level I axillary LNs, ranged from 1.5–2%.
   — There are other studies that have indicated a higher incidence of 'skip' metastases, but this may be due to the difference in definition of Level I vs. Level II axillary LNs.

AXILLARY LYMPH NODE IRRADIATION
[Morrow M, Semin Surg Oncol 12: 321–327, 1996].
[Fisher B, Int J Radiat Oncol Biol Phys 38: 541–550, 1997].
[Singhal H, Breast Cancer Res Treat 37: 50, 1996].
[Vicini FA, Int J Radiat Oncol Biol Phys 39: 1069–1076, 1997].
[Fowble B, 15th Annual International Miami Breast Cancer Conference, February 26–28, 1998].

- Axillary recurrences in ♀ with clinically node(−) breast cancer following total mastectomy, ranges from 21–41% at ∼ 10 years of follow-up.

- [Baxter N, Ann Surg Oncol 3: 235–240, 1996].
  - Factors which correlate with the development of axillary recurrence in ♀ not undergoing an axillary nodal dissection:
    - Age < 65 years old.
    - Tumors > 1.1 cm.
    - Increasing nuclear grade.

- Axillary recurrence rates following axillary sampling or axillary dissection.
  - 15–20% of ♀ who underwent axillary sampling experienced an axillary recurrence at ∼ 7 years of follow-up.
  - ≤ 3% of ♀ who underwent axillary dissection experienced an axillary recurrence at ∼ 7 years of follow-up.

- < 5 axillary LNs is considered an inadequate dissection.

- In the British Columbia and Danish Breast Cancer Group Trials, two prospective Randomized trials:
  - The addition of XRT to axillary sampling ↓ axillary recurrence rates when compared to axillary sampling alone, at ∼ 10 years of follow-up.

- Axillary XRT is indicated for gross extracapsular extension, but not microscopic.

- CONCLUSION:
  - XRT results in regional control rates = surgical dissection in clinically LN(−) ♀.
  - It does not provide prognostic or staging information.

— The ↓ in axillary recurrence rate has in selective patients translated into a modest improvement in survival (4–5%) at ∼ 10 years.

— The use of sentinel node biopsy may eliminate axillary node dissection in ♀ in whom the sentinel node is (−), but axillary dissection will continue to remain important in the treatment of ♀ with (+) sentinel nodes.

● SIDE EFFECTS OF AXILLARY DISSECTION:
[Liljegren G, Eur J Cancer 33: 193–199, 1987].
— Seroma.
— Infection.
— Intercostobrachial nerve syndrome.
— ↓ muscle strength.
— Limited range of motion.
— Arm edema.
— Breast edema.

— Brachial plexopathy and symptomatic pneumonitis are related to the use of a supraclavicular field and occur more often ♀ receiving chemotherapy.

BREAST RECONSTRUCTION AFTER MASTECTOMY

[Harris JR, New Engl J Med 327(6): 390–398, 1992].
[Palm Beach Breast Cancer Conference: An International Symposium,
February 17–19, 1994].

- It is an integral consideration in the management of patients with breast cancer.

- Patient motivation and desire are the main indications for restoring the breast. Immediate reconstruction can generally be offered to patients with stage 0, I and II disease.

- Breast reconstruction can alleviate the sense of deformity that may develop after mastectomy or conservative treatment, i.e. asymmetry of fibrotic breast.

Timing of breast reconstruction

- Immediate reconstruction is oncologically safe and nowadays generally preferred; advantages:
  — Psychological benefits:
    — ↓ fear of mastectomy.
    — ↓ psychological morbidity after mastectomy.
    — Preservation of body image.

  — Aesthetical benefits.

  — Practical benefits:
    — ↓ hospital stay.
    — ↓ number of operations and anaesthesia.
    — ↓ charges.
  — Complication rate is equal to complication rate of mastectomy alone.

- Drawbacks of primary reconstruction are:
  — Team organization.
  — Limited or no histological information.

- Delayed reconstruction:
  — Indication: all stages if uneventful oncological follow-up.
  — Timing: > 6 months following last chemotherapy or XRT.
  — Choice of technique same as primary reconstruction.

- With stage I or II breast cancer reconstruction can be combined with modified radical mastectomy.
  - Usually does not interfere or delay adjuvant chemotherapy unless complications develop.
  - If so, it is usually necessary to delay adjuvant chemotherapy until the wound is healed.

Choice of reconstructive technique

- The most common reconstructions involve implant insertion or transfer of autologous tissue.

- The main goal of breast reconstruction is to obtain symmetry.

- The choice of reconstruction depends on:

  - Oncological considerations.
    - Staging.
    - Tumor grading.
    - Scheduled XRT.

  - Local conditions of the operated breast.
    - Scars.
    - Pectoralis muscle.

- The patient's wishes and concerns about the contralateral breast.
  - Reduction.
  - Augmentation.
  - Mastopexia.
  - Prophylactic mastectomy.

- Surgical skills of the plastic surgeon.

Implants

- The implants (prosthesis, expanders and permanent expandable implants) most often used are constructed of a silicone shell with an interior of silicone gel or saline and are typically placed beneath the pectoralis muscle.

- Tissue expansion also permits breast reconstruction without the need for distant flaps. Expanders distend the remaining pectoralis muscle and skin and need to be replaced after 3–6 months by a definitive implant.
  - Permanent expandable implants avoid a second intervention.
  - Textured surface breast expanders have a lower incidence of capsular contraction and allow late post-operative volume changes.

- Breast reconstruction with implants is an easy and short surgical procedure with few peri-operative complications and does not involve additional scarring at possible donor sites.

- Even in the most positive reports, capsular contracture and implant leakage or rupture are the most frequently encountered problems. The

Literature review of the complications related to breast reconstruction with implants		
	Mean (%)	Range (%)
Capsular contracture	20.9	3.8–55
Wrinkling	12.3	3–26
Skin necrosis	8.5	1.9–22
Implant rupture and deflation	5.9	0–24
Seroma	5.2	1.5–9
Infection	5	0.5–15
Fill port migration and/or failure	4.8	1.6–7
Implant exposure and/or extrusion	4.5	1.5–8
Allergic reactions and/or skin rash	3.1	2.3–3.9
Hematoma	2.5	0–5.8
Displacement	6	—
Gel-bleed, siliconomas	1	—
Implant failure	9.9	1.5–16.6

total number of complications and the limited life span of implants make placement of prostheses a suboptimal choice, especially in younger women.

● There is no scientifically valid evidence to support the association between silicone implants and an increased risk of autoimmune disease. [Gabriel SE, New Engl J Med 336: 677–682, 1997].
  – The U.S. Food and Drug Administration prohibited the use of silicone gel implants in 1992. [Markowitz S, New Engl J Med 326: 713–4, 1992].

● All large demographic studies show no relationship between silicone breast implants and breast cancer.

● Recent studies indicate that the repetitive revisions of implant patients generated higher costs and demands for both the patients and (public) health care insurances on a long-term basis. [Kroll SS et al. Plast Reconstr Surg 97: 364–72, 1996].

● See price comparison table, page 106.

● A natural, soft and warm reconstruction is difficult to obtain with implants, specifically in larger breasts mainly due to a lack of ptosis.

● Indications for implant breast reconstruction:
  – Small sized non-irradiated breasts.
  – ♀ refusing additional scars.
  – ♀ who are not willing or able, due to a poor general condition, to undergo long and extensive surgery.
  – ♀ with limited life expectations (advanced age and poor prognosis).

● In patients requiring chest wall XRT, reconstruction with implants leads to poor results and an unacceptable high rate of complications:
  – XRT ↑ risk of implant failure and capsular contracture.
  – Placing an implant or expander in an irradiated area is very difficult due to tissue fibrosis.
  – Irradiated chest walls are relatively inelastic and are not amenable to tissue expansion.

● Generally, XRT and implants are incompatible.

Autologous tissue

- Despite the increase in surgical complexity, autologous tissue is preferred for breast reconstruction:

  — Avoids implant-related complications.

  — Lower number of procedures and need for future revisions.

  — Autologous methods provide ample amounts of soft, warm and pliable tissues that imitate the normal anatomy more accurately.

  — The long-lasting character of the results and the fact that natural ptosis and the inframammary crease are better defined, add to better cosmetic results and subsequently higher patient satisfaction.

  — The possibility to add supplementary skin to a tight mastectomy scar is a unique feature that avoids overstretching of the skin with subcutaneous expanders.

  — In skin sparing mastectomies the abdominal skin can immediately be used to reconstruct the areola, obviating later reconstructions.

  — In cases of post-mastectomy chest deformities, as, e.g. after radical mastectomy, depressions and contour irregularities can be corrected with the additional tissue of an autologous flap.

  — At the donor site, an aesthetic improvement of the body contour can be achieved by the resection of redundant amounts of fat tissue. This can be an abdominoplasty for the Transverse Rectus Abdominis Myocutaneous (TRAM) flap or a buttock lift for the gluteal flaps.

  — Lower costs are related to autologous tissue mainly due to a ↓ amount of long-term complications and surgical revisions.

  — Volume and shape will follow body weight changes.

  — Spontaneous return of sensation is possible.

  — Offers a valuable solution for partial mastectomies, a problem which is difficult to solve with implants.

– No significant difference in major and minor complication rates compared with the non-autologous methods.

– Autologous tissue is preferred if adjuvant chemo- and/or radiation therapy is expected to be combined in the cancer treatment.

● Most commonly flaps are harvested from the following donor areas:

– Back:
  – The pedicled latissimus dorsi (LD) myocutaneous flap.
  – The thoracodorsal Artery Perforator (TAP) skin-fat flap.

– Abdomen:
  – The pedicled or free transverse rectus abdominis myocutaneous (TRAM) flap.
  – The free Deep Inferior Epigastric Perforator (DIEP) skin-fat flap.

– Buttock:
  – The free superior or inferior Gluteus myocutaneous flap.
  – The free superior gluteal artery perforator (S-GAP) skin-fat flap.

● The TAP, DIEP and S-GAP flaps are recent refinements or 'upgrades' of the conventional myocutaneous back, lower abdominal and gluteal flaps.

– The harvested skin and fat paddles are similar but none of the underlying muscle is sacrificed.

– The preservation of the continuity of the muscle fibers is responsible for a significant decrease in donor site morbidity;

– Normal body movements, strength and in the case of the DIEP flap, the abdominal competence will not be affected and patients can continue with their usual activities of daily living (profession, sports, household, hobbies, etc.) as before their surgery. [Blondeel PhN. Free perforator flaps in breast reconstruction. Ph.D. thesis, Gent, 1998].

● LD and TAP flaps:
  – Safe and relatively simple procedure avoiding microsurgery.
  – Flap is transferred through the axilla in a pedicled fashion.

- Primary indications:
  - Thoracic wall reconstruction.
  - Salvage coverage of exposed implants.
  - Reconstruction of the anterior axillary fold.
  - Reconstruction of a small non-ptotic breast.
  - Partial reconstruction of the outer quadrants after segmentectomy or quadrantectomy.

  - The limited amount of bulk and the unpredictable amount of muscle atrophy often necessitate the placement of implants under the muscle, hereby combining the disadvantages of both techniques.
  - This only applies to the LD flaps.
  - TAP flaps do not require muscle transfer, so there is no muscle atrophy.
  - Long-term data on donor site morbidity after latissimus dorsi muscle harvesting are not yet available, but clinical experience indicates that the impact of resecting the LD muscle does not result in the same degree of morbidity as the TRAM flap.

  - Resection of the muscle does create contour deformity, what is avoided with the TAP flap.

  - Resultant scar on the back is often of poor quality.

- Lower abdominal flaps:
  - First choice as a free flap donor site:
    - Ample amount of lower abdominal fat tissue.
    - Excellent skin quality, texture and colour.
    - Ease of shaping of soft adipose tissue of the abdomen.
    - This procedure should be considered as a first line therapy in women with extra lower abdominal tissue.

  - Pedicled TRAM flap: lower abdominal fat and skin is moved to the chest area and pedicled as a myocutaneous flap on the entire rectus abdominis muscle.
    - The blood supply is based on the superior epigastric vessels, a terminal branch of the internal mammary vessels.

  - Disadvantages:
    - The harvesting of the rectus abdominis muscle causes considerable weakening of the abdominal wall resulting in a decreased abdominal wall competence (bulging and hernias) and strength.

— Epigastric bulging.
— Ill-defined inframammary crease.
— High number of partial flap necrosis and fat necroses.

— Increased flow to the TRAM flap can be obtained by designing it with some perforators above the umbilicus, with a bipedicled TRAM flap and possibly with delay. The use of vascular delay of the TRAM flap for ~ 2 weeks before the breast reconstruction can enhance blood flow and avoid venous congestion in the flap (Fig. 10).

— Bipedicled TRAM flap: have an increased vascularization and have been shown to be safer when there are specific risk factors, i.e. obesity and cigarette smoking. Nevertheless the harvesting of both rectus muscles should be avoided as much as possible.

— The free TRAM flap: same skin paddle as the pedicled TRAM, but the flap is now vascularised by the deep inferior epigastric vessels, that are cut at the external iliac vessels before transfer to the chest. An arterial and venous micro-anastomosis is then performed to recipient vessels in the axilla or to the internal mammary vessels. [Schusterman MA, Ann Plast Surg 32: 234–241, 1994].

— The free TRAM is better vascularised by the larger deep inferior epigastric vessels and requires less muscle dissection and harvesting, resulting in a lower partial necrosis rate, reduced abdominal discomfort and less donor site morbidity.

— The operative technique of a free TRAM flap is more demanding and operative time is increased. Additionally, the viability of the flap is based entirely on the success of the microvascular anastomosis, what in rare cases of failure can lead to total flap loss.

— The superb cosmetic results and the lower total complication rate justify the use of the free TRAM over the pedicled TRAM.

— Usually requires a 5–7 day hospitalisation and a 2–3 month recovery period.

— Abdominal closure, often with Prolene mesh is necessary to give a tight abdominal wall and avoid post-operative hernia.

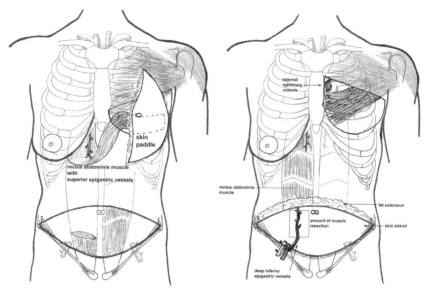

Fig. 10. Schematic overview of the surgical differences between the pedicled (left) and the free (right) TRAM flap.

— Despite the reduced amount of muscle resection, decreased abdominal wall competence (umbilical and abdominal asymmetry, bulging and hernia) and strength affects daily living activities in 20–30% of patients, especially if they are physically active. [Blondeel PhN. Br J Plast Surg 50: 315–21, 1997].

— Free DIEP flap:
  — Same skin paddle as the pedicled TRAM, but without harvesting any muscle at all.
  — The blood vessels travelling through the muscle from deeper layers towards the skin, the so-called 'perforators' are dissected free from the surrounding rectus abdominis muscle.
  — The splitting of the muscle in the direction of the muscle fibers around the perforating vessels allowed selective harvesting of the flap and its vessels, and preservation of muscle continuity, vascularization and motor innervation. [Blondeel PhN. Br J Plast Surg 47:495–501, 1994].
  — Pure sensate nerves can also be isolated and harvested with the flap to restore sensation in the reconstructed breast (Fig. 11).

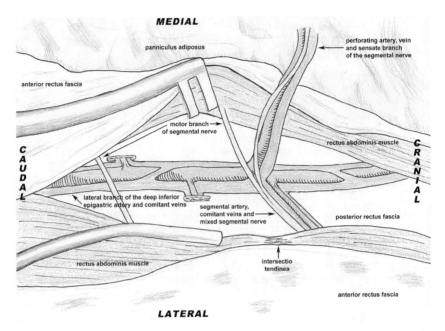

MEDIAL

panniculus adiposus

perforating artery, vein
and sensate branch
of the segmental nerve

anterior rectus fascia

motor branch
of segmental nerve

rectus abdominis muscle

C
A
U
D
A
L

C
R
A
N
I
A
L

lateral branch of the deep inferior
epigastric artery and comitant veins

segmental artery,
comitant veins and
mixed segmental nerve

posterior rectus fascia

rectus abdominis muscle

intersectio
tendinea

anterior rectus fascia

LATERAL

Fig. 11. Schematic drawing of the anatomical relationships between vessels and nerves at the level of a lateral perforator in the lower third of the abdominal wall on the left side.

– A prospective study indicated less umbilical and abdominal asymmetry, bulging and hernias, limited decrease of rectus muscle power, intact function of the oblique muscles and preservation of normal trunk movements in activities of daily life [Blondeel PhN. Br J Plast Surg 50: 322–30, 1997].

– Besides the minimal donor site morbidity, the free DIEP flap maintains the well-known advantages of the TRAM flap and discards its disadvantages.
  – The long vascular pedicle facilitates flap shaping and positioning.
  – Less post-operative pain allows early mobilisation and swift rehabilitation resulting in a decreased hospital stay. [Blondeel PhN. Free perforator flaps in breast reconstruction. Ph.D. thesis, Gent, 1998].
  – The main disadvantages of a perforator flap are the steep learning curve, the need for tedious dissection and the prolonged operating time.

- The free DIEP flap demonstrates comparable complication rates as the free TRAM flap, making the DIEP flap a safe and reliable technique (Figs. 12–14).

● Gluteal flaps.

- The superior- and inferior-myocutaneous gluteal free flaps have been considered as valuable alternatives to the latissimus dorsi or TRAM flap since 1975. [Fujino T. Plast Reconstr Surg 56: 178–81, 1975].

- Advantages:
  - Coverage of the scars by normal underwear.
  - Less donor morbidity compared to TRAM flaps.
  - Availability of generous amounts of tissue, even in thin persons.
  - Improved projection of the reconstructed breast.

- Disadvantages:
  - Low quality scar and contour defect.

  - Superior gluteal flap:
    - Short vascular pedicle and difficult dissection due to its poor intra-operative exposure.

- Inferior gluteal flap:
  - Exposed the femoral cutaneous- and sciatic nerve leading to paresthesias and pain syndromes in the lower limb.

  - The relatively short pedicle of both flaps necessitated vascular anastomosis to the internal mammary vessels or the use of vein grafts to the axillary vessels.

  - The firmer consistency of gluteal fat, the smaller skin paddle compared to TRAM or DIEP flaps and the absence of sensate reinnervation were other arguments to turn this flap into a second choice.

- Gluteal flaps are indicated in patients with an asthenic body habitus or with excessive abdominal scarring.

- The S-GAP flap is the ultimate upgrade of this myocutaneous flap as no gluteus maximus muscle is harvested.

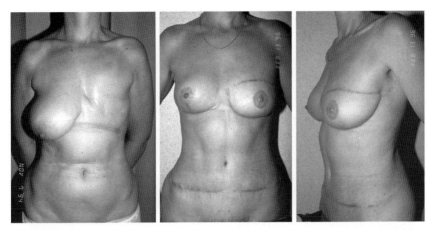

Fig. 12. The pre-operative (left) and 15 months post-operative views of a 41 yr old woman who has undergone secondary breast reconstruction with a free DIEP flap on the left side in the first phase, nipple reconstruction and right breast reduction after 7 months, and finally tattoo of the nipple-areolar complex 10 weeks later.

— The flap is vascularised by one single perforator originating from the superior gluteal artery.
— The development of the S-GAP flap in breast reconstruction by Allen and Tucker avoided unnecessary resection of gluteus maximus muscle, created increased pedicle length and improved intra-operative exposure. [Allen RJ. Plast Reconstr Surg 95: 1207–12, 1995].
— The perforators of the superior instead of the inferior gluteal artery are preferred to harvest the gluteal tissue.

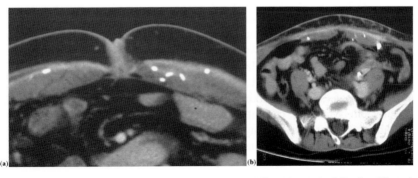

Fig. 13. (a) Axial CT-scan images, at the level of the umbilicus 6 months following bilateral DIEP flap harvesting, show normal-sized rectus abdominis muscles with vascular clips within each muscle. (b) A second cross-section 4 cm lower with the same findings.

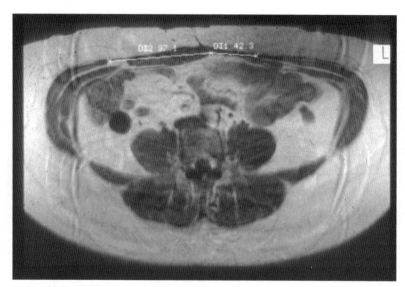

Fig. 14. Horizontal MRI cut at the level of the umbilicus (▽) of a unilateral free TRAM flap patient. The muscle was harvested on the left side.

— The ability to restore the sensate innervation of the flap adds another advantage to the S-GAP flap. The superior buttock nerves or 'nervi clunium superiores' originate in the dorsal branches of the lumbar segmental nerves and can be harvested in selected cases. [Blondeel PhN. Free perforator flaps in breast reconstruction. Ph.D. thesis, Gent, 1998].

— The free sensate superior gluteal artery perforator flap is a valuable alternative for autologous breast reconstruction if lower abdominal adipose tissue is not available and is a better option than the free myocutaneous gluteal flap (Fig. 15).

● The goal of the breast reconstruction is to match the opposite breast. If sufficient symmetry cannot be reached, corrective surgery of the contralateral breast (breast augmentation, reduction, mastopexia, etc.) can be performed about 6 months later.

Nipple-areolar reconstruction
● Usually performed as a separate procedure, 6 months after the breast reconstruction when there is satisfactory breast symmetry (Fig. 16).

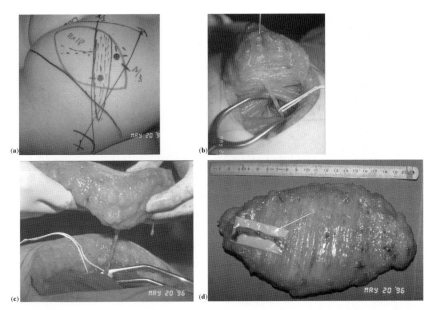

Fig. 15. (a) Flap markings of the free S-GAP flap (red lines); the black dots indicate two perforators located by the unidirectional Doppler flowmetry, the shaded area indicates the position of the piriformis muscle; (b,c) the free S-GAP flap at the donor site with its perforator (arrow) still connected to the SGA; (d) after transsecting the vascular pedicle a free skin flap is obtained without any muscle.

Breast reconstruction and oncology
[Noone RB, Plast Reconstr Surg 93: 96–106, 1994].

- The biology of breast cancer is not altered by breast reconstruction.

- Breast reconstruction does not compromise adequate cancer treatment.

- Immediate breast reconstruction does not increase the rate of local recurrences or secondary primary cancers and does not alter the disease free interval and patient survival.

- Immediate breast reconstruction does not interfere with the detection of local recurrence, nor does it increase the incidence of local failures.

- Immediate breast reconstruction does not delay adjuvant therapy.

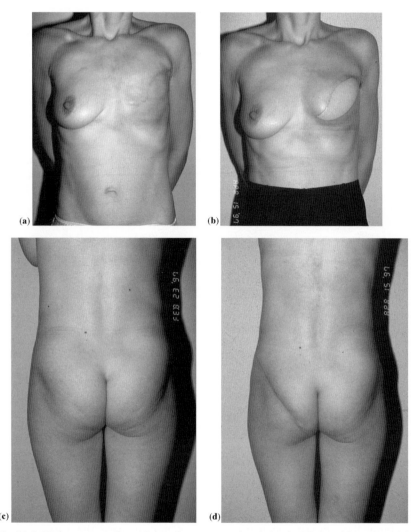

Fig. 16. (a,b) the pre-operative and 6 weeks post-operative views of a 36 year old woman (with a BMI of 18,7) after unilateral secondary breast reconstruction with a free S-GAP flap; (c,d) the pre-operative and 6 months post-operative views of the donor area.

- Reconstructions do not interfere with the treatment of local, regional or distant metastases.

- The need for postoperative systemic therapy should not be considered a contraindication to immediate reconstruction.

— RT and implants are incompatible.
— Chemotherapy and XRT can be started early if no major Complications and normal wound healing occur.

● Good post-reconstruction follow-up is possible with non-imaging and imaging techniques. Important factors are:
— Patient awareness of symptoms and self-examination.
— Physician's clinical examination.
— Clinical laboratory.
— Correlation of physical findings, surgical procedure and imaging procedure.

● In case of doubt: excisional biopsy.

GENERAL FACTS ABOUT BREAST CANCER AND CHEMO-HORMONAL THERAPY

- Prognostic factors:
  - Lymph node status.
    - LN(−) breast cancer recurs later than LN(+).
  - Estrogen receptor (ER) status.
    - ER(+) patients have higher survival rates.
    - Most likely postmenopausal.
  - Age.
    - ♀ < 35 and > 75 years old at presentation have a worse prognosis.
    - ♀ < 35 years old have a higher incidence of local breast recurrence than older patients.

- Adjuvant treatment:
  - Adjuvant chemotherapy or tamoxifen are of benefit in many patients with stage I/II breast cancer.
  - Adjuvant chemotherapy has shown most benefit in premenopausal patients with 1–3 (+)LN.
  - Ideal regimen not known (CMF, CAF).
  - Adriamycin is believed to be the most active single agent.
  - Adriamycin in some sort of regimen is standard, but no data to document superior efficacy vs. less toxic regimens.

Overall therapy				
	Premenopausal		Postmenopausal	
	ER +	ER −	ER +	ER −
Negative nodes	Chemo and/or Tamox.	Chemo	Tamox ± Chemo (NSABP-B20 suggests Chemo + Tamox)	Chemo and/or Tamox
Positive nodes	Chemo ± Tamox.	Chemo	Tamox ± Chemo (NSABP-B16 and Meta-analysis suggests Chemo + Tamox)	Chemo and/or Tamox

PRIMARY CHEMOTHERAPY
[Veronesi U, Ann Surg 222: 612–618, 1995].
[Smith IE, J Clin Oncol 13: 424–429, 1995].
[Bonadonna G, CA Cancer J 45: 227–243, 1995].
[Harris JR, New Engl J Med 327(6): 390–398, 1992].

- Primary chemotherapy, also known as neo-adjuvant or pre-operative chemotherapy.

- Introduced 25 years ago.

- Advantages:
  - ↓ tumor size and ↑ the possibility of breast conservation.
    - Avoid mastectomy if possible.
  - ↑ effectiveness of systemic treatment by attempting to reach micrometastatic disease at its most sensitive phase.
  - ↓ any possible stimulation or leakage of metastatic cancer cells by excising the tumor.
  - May turn off surgically induced growth factors.
  - ↑ ability to evaluate chemoresponsiveness of the tumor.

- Disadvantages:
  - ↓ ability of the surgeon to identify the original tumor site when the tumor is no longer palpable.
    - Accurate estimation of tumor size in the operating room is crucial for deciding the type and extent of operation to be performed.
  - ↓ ability to evaluate axillary node status.
  - ↓ ability to evaluate biologic characteristics of tumor.
  - Therapy is not tailored to patients individually, based on post-surgical prognostic indicators.

- Surgical pitfalls:
  [Zurrida S, Eur J Surg Oncol 20: 641–3, 1994].
  - Location and size of tumor mass should be tattooed on the skin surface before beginning therapy.
  - 3 weeks after the last chemotherapy cycle, each patient should be clinically and mammographically evaluated.
  - When microcalcifications are observed in the initial mammogram, specimen mammography should be performed to ensure that the whole lesion is removed.

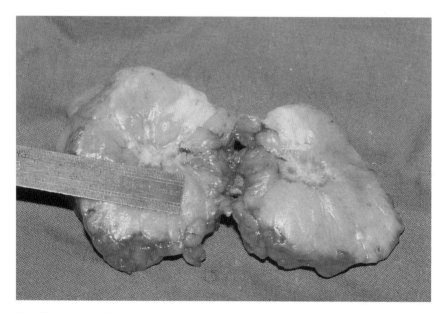

Fig. 17. Intraoperative measurement of tumor diameter and of healthy surrounding tissue (imperative after neoadjuvant chemotherapy).

— The final decision on which surgery to perform should be taken in the operating room after careful evaluation of tumor regression, resection margins, tumor/breast size ratio and the extent of microcalcifications (Fig. 17).

- NSABP-B18.
  [Kalaycioglu M, Proc Am Soc Clin Oncol 13: 65 (A64) 1994].
  [Fisher B, J Clin Oncol 15: 2483–2493, 1997].
  — 1523 ♀ with stage I/II breast cancer.
  — Randomized to: pre-operative doxorubicin/cyclophosphamide
  vs.
  post-operative doxorubicin/cyclophosphamide.
  — All patients in both groups received doxorubicin and cyclophosphamide (AC) therapy every 21 days at 60 and 600 mg/m^2, respectively, for four courses.
  — 60% of the tumors were between 2 and 5 cm in size.
  — All patients > 50 years old began tamoxifen 20 mg/day at the completion of chemotherapy.
  — 747 eligible patients received pre-operative AC.

— 759 eligible patients received post-operative AC.
— 4-year follow-up data.
— RESULTS:

   — In 80% of the patients after pre-operative therapy, breast tumor size was reduced by $\geq 50\%$, regardless of the initial size of the tumor.

   — 36% had a clinical CR.

   — 26% of ♀ with a clinical CR had a pathologic CR.

   — Clinical nodal response occurred in 89% of LN(+) patients.

   — Multivariate analysis indicated that clinical tumor size (smaller tumors) and clinical nodal status (+ nodes) were independent predictors of complete clinical response in the breast.
      — Age (younger patients) was of borderline significance.

   — Overall 12% more lumpectomies were performed in the pre-operative group and in ♀ with tumors ≥ 5.1 cm, there was a 175% increase in number of lumpectomies.

   — DFS is identical in both groups.

   — OS is identical in both groups.

● The Bordeaux Study.
   [Mauriac L, Annals of Oncology 2: 347–354, 1991].
   — Randomized, single institution study.
   — 272 ♀ with operable breast cancer.
   — Randomized to surgery or chemotherapy prior to surgery.
   — T > 3 cm by clinical examination.
   — Patients assessed for metastatic disease by bone scan, liver function tests and chest X-ray.

   — Group I:
      — 138 patients treated initially with mastectomy and LN dissection.
      — LN(+) or ER/PR(−) patients were treated with adjuvant chemotherapy.
      — LN(−) and ER/PR(+) patients received no further therapy.

— Group II:
— 134 patients treated initially with chemotherapy.
— Chemotherapy was followed by loco-regional treatment:
— Mastectomy was done if residual tumor was > 2 cm.
— Lumpectomy with LN dissection and XRT was done if residual tumor was < 2 cm.
  — Radiation alone was done in patients with complete responses.
  — XRT included the breast, axilla, internal mammary nodes and supraclavicular area.
  — 50 Gy was given to the breast with 20 Gy boost.

— The same chemotherapy was used in both groups.
  — Three cycles of:
    — Epirubicin 50 mg/m^2.
    — Vincristine 1 mg/m^2.
    — Methotrexate 20 mg/m^2.
  — Followed by three cycles of:
    — Mitomycin C (Mutamycin) 10 mg/m^2.
    — Thiotepa 20 mg/m^2.
    — Vindesine 4 mg/m^2.

— Patients in both groups were identical with respect to age, hormonal status and tumor size.

— Median follow-up of ~ 34 months.

— Local recurrences were more frequent in Group II (initial chemotherapy).

— Better overall survival in Group II (initial chemotherapy) ($P = 0.04$).

— CONCLUSION:
  — Induction chemotherapy can be proposed to ♀ who prefer to conserve their breast.
  — With a 50–70% chance of undergoing conservative treatment.

— Problem with study:
  — The treatment arms were not really balanced.

● Milan Trials.

Bonadonna and Veronesi [Bonadonna G, Lancet 341(June 5): 1485, 1993].

— The first preoperative chemotherapy Milan trial.

— 227 ♀, with T ≥ 3 cm, candidates for mastectomy, were randomized.

— Median age: 49 years.

— Patients with fixation or direct extension into the chest wall were excluded.

— Primary chemotherapy was administered:
  1. CMF (cyclophosphamide/methotrexate/fluorouracil)
  2. FAC (fluorouracil/doxorubicin/cyclophosphamide)
  3. FEC (fluorouracil/epirubicin/cyclophosphamide)
  4. FNC (fluorouracil/novantrone/cyclophosphamide)
  5. Adriamycin 75–90 mg/m^2

— Outline of trial.

Diagnosis.

↓

3–4 cycles of chemotherapy.

↓

T < 3 cm (220 ♀) → Quadrantectomy + axillary dissection + XRT (60 Gy)

T > 3 cm (19 ♀) → MRM + axillary dissection

↓

LN(+) or LN(−)/ER(−) → 2–3 more cycles of chemotherapy

LN(−)/ER(+) → no more therapy.

— 78% of patients showed complete or partial response, 15% showed minor response, and 3% experienced progressive disease.

— Tumor shrinkage to < 3 cm was documented in 83% of the 220 women subjected to surgery.

— Conservative surgery was feasible in 91% of the patients.

— Tumor response was unrelated to age, menopausal status, drug regimen used, or number of treatment cycles.

— The frequency of response was greater in receptor (−) tumors.

— 8 ♀ achieved CR with (−)LN in the axilla.
  — At 3 years, 7 out of 8 ♀ remain alive and free of disease.
  — 1 out of 8 ♀ relapsed in the CNS.

— CONCLUSION:
  — Full-dose primary chemotherapy sequentially combined with conservative surgery and XRT can offer an effective and safe alternative to mastectomy.

● Second preoperative chemotherapy Milan Trial.

  Bonadonna [Bonadonna G, Proc Am Soc Clin Oncol 13: 107 (A230) 1994].
  — 210 ♀ with T > 2.5 cm (median 4 cm).
  — Doxorubicin was given alone q 3 weeks × three cycles.
  — Clinical response rate → 12%.
    — Response rate was lower than in the first preoperative Milan trial which was 21%.
    — The overall response rate was similar for both studies.
    — Only 3% of patients in either study showed tumor progression while on chemotherapy.

  — Following the preoperative chemotherapy the same surgical steps outlined in the first trial were followed.

  — In patients responding to primary chemotherapy, the cellular features of the residual tumor were in general very similar to the cellular features of the initial biopsy.
    — Extensive necrosis was never found.
    — Occasional necrotic foci were detected.

  — In the first study, XRT was delivered concurrently with adjuvant (postoperative) chemotherapy.

  — In the second study, XRT was delivered at the end of the adjuvant (postoperative) chemotherapy.
  — Adjuvant chemotherapy was delivered as in the first trial.
  — Final results and analyses are pending.

● The role of taxanes in pre-operative chemotherapy has yet to be determined.

- NSABP-B27.
  - Ongoing trial.
  - Cytologically or histologically proven breast cancer (tumor in place).
  - Clinically T_{1-3}; N_{0-1}.
  - 1000 ♀ randomized to 1 of 3 arms of preoperative chemotherapy.
    - AC + TAM → Surgery

         vs.

      AC + TAM → Taxotere → Surgery

         vs.

      AC + TAM → Surgery → Taxotere.

STAGE III DISEASE
[Perez EA, Oncology 11 (suppl 9): 9–17, 1997]
- Stage IIIA/B patients have a high incidence of local relapse following mastectomy alone.
  - Stage IIIA -locally advanced breast cancer.
    - T_3, N_1 or any N_2.
  - Stage IIIB -inflammatory breast cancer.
    - Any N_3 or any T_4.

- The probability of distant metastases is high. For these reasons both radiotherapy and systemic chemotherapy are employed.

- In most clinical trials 3–4 four cycles of a doxorubicin-containing regimen before surgery will reduce the tumor size and facilitate local ablation in > 80% of the cases.

- Clinical complete remissions have been reported in 10–20% of patients.

- Only 2/3rds of the patients with a clinical CR will have a pathologic CR.

- [McCready DR, Arch Surg 124: 21–25, 1989].
  - On multivariate analysis the number of (+)LN's found after induction chemotherapy proved to be the best predictor of both relapse and death.

- Then radiation or surgery, usually mastectomy, is followed by further chemotherapy.

- Combined systemic approach.
  - Significantly improves survival.
  - 3-year survival rates range from 50–80%.
  - 5-year survival rates range from 50–60%.
  - Median survival is ~ 3–4 years.
  - The optimal timing and sequencing of the combined modality approach including chemotherapy, surgery, and XRT have yet to be determined.

- [High Risk Breast Cancer. Berlin. Springer, 1991 pp. 382–415].
  - Three cycles of induction chemotherapy with FAC (fluorouracil, adriamycin, Cyclophosphamide) followed by mastectomy, six post-

operative cycles of adjuvant chemotherapy (FAC), and finally radiation therapy to the chest wall.
— The 10-year overall survival for stage IIIA disease was 56%.
— The 10-year overall survival for stage IIIB disease was 26%.

- Pre-operative chemotherapy in Pre-operative chemotherapy in locally advanced breast cancer.
  — French Study.
  [Scholl SM, Eur J Cancer 30A: 645–652, 1994].
    — Tumors > 3 cm.
    — 390 premenopausal ♀ randomized prospectively:
      — Pre-operative chemotherapym — FAC × 4 → XRT → surgery.
                          vs.
      — XRT → surgery → post-operative chemotherapy FAC × 4.
    — Median follow-up 54 months.
    — Statistically significant survival difference favored the pre-operative chemotherapy arm.
      — 5-year survival rate 90 vs. 80%.
    — There was no local recurrence rate difference noted among the two treatment groups.
  — NSABP-B18.
  [Fisher B, J Clin Oncol 15: 2483–2493, 1997].
    — For further details, please refer to the Primary Chemotherapy section on page 83.
    — 1523 ♀ randomized.
      — Pre-operative AC × four cycles vs.
      — Post-operative AC × four cycles.
    — 4-year follow-up data for both treatment groups:
      — Equivalent DFS.
      — Equivalent OS.
    — 12% more lumpectomies were performed in the pre-operative arm.

- The impact of newer chemotherapeutic agents such as taxanes, and high-dose chemotherapy with stem cell transplantation, on stage III disease remains to be determined.

- Inflammatory breast cancer.
  [Jiyesimi IA, J Clin Oncol 10: 1014–1024, 1992].
    — A rapid onset of disease (< 3 months) is often used to differentiate inflammatory breast cancer from locally advanced breast cancer.

- Before the use of combined-modality therapy in this disease, the 5 year survival rates were < 5%.
- There are no randomized trials in the treatment of this disease, however the data suggest that the combined systemic approach prolongs survival.
- With combined-modality therapy, ~ 35% remain disease free at 10 years.
- Late relapses of inflammatory breast cancer are uncommon.
- Because inflammatory breast cancer is often diffuse, breast conserving surgery is not a practical option.
- Mastectomy immediately after the diagnosis of inflammatory breast carcinoma should rarely if ever be done.
- Intra-arterial cytotoxic chemotherapy.
  [Chang HT, Am J Clin Oncol 20(5): 493–499, 1997].
  [Stephens FO, Lancet (30 Aug): 435–438, 1980].
  [Stephens FO, Cancer 66: 645–650, 1980].
  - Intra-arterial cytotoxic chemotherapy can obtain high response rate and quick tumor reduction.
  - After the 'first pass effect' in the body region bearing the tumor, the intra-arterial chemotherapy may be equal to systemic treatment against distant metastases.
  - May even be beneficial as first line therapy.
    [Noguchi S, Cancer 61: 1483–1491, 1988].
  - ↓ tumor size and cutaneous inflammatory response.

ADJUVANT CHEMOTHERAPY IN PREMENOPAUSAL BREAST CANCER
[Hortobagyi GN, CA Cancer J Clin 45: 199–226, 1995].

- Micrometastatic disease is present in ~ 25–30% of LN(−) patients and 35–90% of LN(+) patients.
  - Chemotherapy is used in an attempt to eliminate micrometastases.

- NSABP-B01.
  [Fisher B, Surg Gynecol Obstet 140: 528–534, 1975].
  - First randomized clinical trial conducted by NSABP.
  - On the day of mastectomy, patients were randomized to:
    - Thiotepa, that day and on each of the first two post-op days
      vs.
      PLACEBO.

  - CONCLUSIONS:
    - DFS and OS could be significantly improved by chemotherapy.
    - Response to chemotherapy was heterogeneous.

- NSABP-B05.
  [Fisher B, New Engl J Med 292: 117–122, 1975].
  - ♀ Randomized to:
    - Melphalan (Alkeran)(L-PAM) × 5 days q 6 weeks × 2 years
      vs.
      PLACEBO.

  - CONCLUSION:
    - Significant benefit of chemotherapy to premenopausal ♀s with node(+) disease.

- Milan I.
  [Bonadonna G, New Engl J Med 332: 901–906, 1995].
  - Bonadonna's original study, 1973–75.
    - 386 premenopausal patients.
    - 20-year follow-up.
  - CMF vs. observation after radical mastectomy.
  - Treated with CMF × 1 year (p.o. Cytoxan).
    vs.
    OBSERVATION.

- The CMF group benefited significantly from chemotherapy.
  - Premenopausal 1–3 (+)LN.
  - Improved overall survival and relapse free survival.
  - Median survival for control arm (no chemo) → 8 years (at 8 years > 50% dead).
  - Median survival for chemotherapy arm reached at 18 years, at least a 10-year benefit for patients receiving > 85% of the optimal chemotherapy dose.

- Overview analysis.
  [EBCTCG, Lancet 339: 1–15, 1992].
  [EBCTCG, Lancet 339: 71–85, 1992].
  - Chemotherapy vs. no chemotherapy.
  - Evaluated 26000 ♀ receiving chemotherapy for 1 year.
  - From U.S. and Europe.
  - Meta-analyses usually do not identify the following:
    - Dose intensity.
    - Dose sequencing and selection.
    - Population differences.

- CONCLUSIONS:
  - Six months of chemotherapy as good as one year (usually CMF).
  - Clear benefit, if < 50 years.
  - 5-year survival 72.8 vs. 65.9% in ♀ < 50 years of age.
  - Combination chemotherapy is better than single agent chemotherapy.
  - Few Anthracycline-based studies were included, so no substantial conclusion could be drawn regarding these regimens.
  - Adjuvant chemotherapy in premenopausal ♀ especially with (+) LN → provides improved relapse free survival and Improved overall survival.
  - Adjuvant chemotherapy in postmenopausal ♀, provides 3–4% overall improvement.
  - Survival benefit from chemotherapy was greater at 10 years than at 5 years.
  - Major finding: Relative reductions in mortality risk were the same for LN(−) and LN(+) ♀.

- Ovarian ablation—Oxford Overview Study.
  [EBCTCG, Lancet 348(9036): 1189–1196, 1996].

- 1817 evaluable ♀ were randomized in 12 trials before 1980.
- 934 ♀ had ovarian ablation by surgery or XRT.
- Menopausal status was not consistently defined across the trials.
- In ♀ < 50 years of age, ovarian suppression as sole adjuvant treatment, reduces the annual risk of death by almost 30%, at 15 years. (similar to the benefit obtained with adjuvant chemotherapy; however, there is much less experience with oophorectomy than with chemotherapy).
- The benefit was significant for both LN(+) and LN(−) ♀.

● NSABP-B11.
  [Fisher B, J Clin Oncol 7: 572–582, 1989].
  - Premenopausal and PR(−) postmenopausal ♀ (TAM-nonresponsive).
  - Randomized to receive.
    - PAF vs. PF.
      - P = L-PAM.
      - A = doxorubicin.
      - F = fluorouracil.
  - 6-year follow-up.

  - CONCLUSION:
    - DFS and OS significantly better in doxorubicin arm.

● Bonadonna.
  [Buzzoni R, J Clin Oncol 9: 2134–2140, 1991].
  - 359 ♀ all with four or more (+)LN.
  - One third had > 10 (+)LN.
  - Two thirds were premenopausal.
  - Randomized 2–4 weeks after surgery to receive one of two chemotherapy regimens.
  - Half received mastectomy and half were treated with lumpectomy + axillary LN dissection, followed by XRT.
  - XRT was 50 Gy + 10 Gy boost, 6–8 weeks after the surgery, given concurrently with chemotherapy.
  - 179 ♀ received adriamycin followed by CMF.
  - 180 ♀ received alternating adriamycin and CMF.

Regimens

Group I: A,A,A,A,CMF,CMF,CMF,CMF,CMF,CMF,CMF,CMF

vs.

Group II: A,CMF,CMF,A,CMF,CMF,A,CMF,CMF,A,CMF,CMF

- All cycles given q 3 weeks.
- Both groups received same total dose, however the group with adriamycin first did better.
  - Adriamycin 75 mg/m^2 IV.
  - Cyclophosphamide 600 mg/m^2 IV.
  - Methotrexate 40 mg/m^2 IV.
  - 5-fluorouracil 600 mg/m^2 IV.

- CONCLUSION:
  - 5-year relapse-free survival was superior with the Group I regimen.
    - 61 vs. 38% ($P = 0.001$).
  - 5-year overall survival was superior with the Group I regimen.
    - 78 vs. 62% ($P = 0.005$).

- NSABP-B13.
  [Fisher, B, New Engl J Med 320: 473–478, 1989].
  [Margolese R, J Natl Cancer Inst Monogr 11: 41–48, 1992].
  [Fisher B, J Clin Oncol 14(7): 1982–1992, 1996].
  - 760 ER($-$), LN($-$) pre/postmenopausal ♀ were randomized after surgery:
    - Chemotherapy vs. observation alone.
  - 32% of patients were treated with breast conservation surgery and XRT.
  - The chemotherapy used was sequential methotrexate (M) 100 mg/m^2 i.v. bolus and fluorouracil (F) 600 mg/m^2 i.v. bolus, 1 h after M on day 1 and day 8 of each cycle. (M → F).
  - The chemotherapy was followed by leucovorin 10 mg/m^2 q 6 h x 6 doses and it was to begin 24 h after M.
  - Therapy was given q 4 weeks × 12 cycles.
  - 732 patients were eligible for follow-up.
  - Median follow-up 8 years.
  - 74% of chemotherapy-arm patients were free of disease vs. 59% in the observation-arm ($P < 0.001$).
  - Benefit in disease free survival occurred in both pre and post-menopausal ♀.
    - Benefit in DFS ♀ ≤ 49 years of age, who received M → F: 69 vs. 56% in observation arm ($P = 0.006$).
    - Among ♀ ≥ 50 years of age, the benefit was 81 vs. 63%, respectively ($P = 0.002$).
  - A survival advantage was evident in older patients: 89 vs. 80% ($P = 0.03$).

- NSABP-B19.
  [Fisher B, J Clin Oncol 14(7): 1982–1992, 1996].
  - 1095 ER(−)/LN(−) pre/postmenopausal ♀ were Randomized.
  - CMF chemotherapy vs. M → F.
  - 1074 patients were eligible for follow-up.
  - The chemotherapy was administered for six cycles instead of 12 as in NSABP-B13.
  - CMF was administered as follows:
    - Cyclophosphamide (100 mg/m^2) p.o. q day, days 1–14, q 28 days × 6 cycles.
    - Methotrexate (40 mg/m^2) i.v. day 1 and day 8, q 28 days × 6 cycles.
    - Fluorouracil (600 mg/m^2) i.v. day 1 and day 8, q 28 days × 6 cycles.
  - All other aspects of the administration of therapy were similar to NSABP-B13.
  - Mean follow-up: 5 years.
  - Benefit in DFS (82 vs. 73%; $P < 0.001$) and a borderline survival advantage (88 vs. 85%; $P = 0.06$), were evident in the CMF arm.
  - The DFS (84 vs. 72%; $P < 0.001$) and survival benefit (89 vs. 84%; $P = 0.04$) from CMF were greater in ♀ ≤ 49 years of age.

- NSABP-B23 (ongoing trial).
  - ∼ 2000 patients, LN(−), ER/PR(−).
  - Pre/postmenopausal women.
  - AC vs. CMF, followed by tamoxifen 10 mg b.i.d. vs. placebo.
  - AC vs. CMF, has been previously looked at in LN(+) patients and felt to be equivocal (NSABP-B15).

- [Henderson IC, Proc Am Soc Clin Oncol 17: A390, 1998].
  - Ongoing trial
  - 3170 ♀ with primary operable LN(+) breast cancer.

  - Randomized to:
    Post-operative adjuvant chemotherapy.
    Cyclophosphamide + Adriamycin (AC) ± Paclitaxel q 3 weeks × 4.
    Group I.   C 600 mg/m^2 and A 60 mg/m^2.
    Group II. C 600 mg/m^2 and A 75 mg/m^2.
    Group III. C 600 mg/m^2 and A 90 mg/m^2 + G-CSF.
  - Each group was further Randomized into concurrent Paclitaxel or no Paclitaxel.

— Paclitaxel was given at a dose of 175 mg/m² over 3 hours.
— ♀ with ER(+) tumors had the option of taking tamoxifen 20 mg/day × 5 years.
— Median follow-up is 18 months.

— Preliminary RESULTS:
  — Disease free survival.
    — AC + Paclitaxel → 90%.
    — AC alone → 86%.
  — Overall survival.
    — AC + Paclitaxel → 97%.
    — AC alone → 95%.

— SIDE EFFECTS of AC + T:
  — Myelsuppression 21%.
  — Neuropathy 5%.
  — Pain 5%.
  — Hyperglycemia 5%.
  — Post-chemotherapy cardiotoxicity 6%.

Chemotherapy dose intensity

● CALGB 8541.
  [Budman DR, J Natl Cancer Inst 90: 1205–1211, 1998].
  [Wood WC, New Engl J Med 330(18): 1253–1259, 1994].
  — 1550 stage II breast cancer patients were randomized and evaluable.
  — LN(+), ER(+) or ER(−) breast cancer.
  — Tamoxifen × 5 years, only given to ER(+) postmenopausal women.
  — Tamoxifen administered after chemotherapy.
  — The high-dose and moderate-dose arms received the same total dose but different dose intensities.

  — Follow-up 9 years.
    — Significant improvement in disease-free survival ($P < 0.001$) and overall survival ($P = 0.0034$) in high-dose arm vs. low dose arm.
    — Marginally better survival in high-dose arm vs. medium dose arm.
    — Overall 5-year survival.
      — 72% for low-dose arm.
      — 77% for moderate-dose arm.
      — 78% for high-dose arm.

	High-dose mg/m^2 × 4 months	Medium-dose mg/m^2 × 6 months	Low-dose mg/m^2 × 4 months
Cyclophosphamide Day 1	600	400	300
Doxorubicin Day 1	60	40	30
Fluorouracil Days 1 & 8	600	400	300
Number of ♀ in group	519	513	518

— Dose reduction should be generally avoided in the adjuvant setting.

— See Prognostic Factors section concerning interaction of C-erbB-2 gene and dose intensity.
   — ♀ with c-erbB-2 over-expression had a 60% improved outcome with a high-dose doxorubicin regimen.

- NSABP-B22.
  [Dimitrov N, Proc Am Soc Clin Oncol 13: 64 (A58) 1994].
  — Evaluation of dose intensity and increasing total dose of cyclophosphamide.
  — 2300 operable, LN(+) breast cancer ♀ Randomized.
  — All ♀ ≥ 50 years old received tamoxifen 10 mg p.o. b.i.d. starting on day 1 of chemotherapy × 5 years.

Dose intense cyclophosphamide			
	Group I	Group II	Group III
Adriamycin (A)	60 mg/m^2 q 21 d × 4	60 mg/m^2 q 21 d × 4	60 mg/m^2 q 21 d × 4
Cyclophosphamide (C)	600 mg/m^2 q 21 d × 4	1200 mg/m^2 q 21 d × 2	1200 mg/m^2 q 21 d × 4

— All three groups received the same dose of adriamycin 60 mg/m^2 i.v. on day 1 q 3 weeks × 4.

— RESULTS:
— No difference in DFS or OS between pre and postmenopausal ♀.
— No difference DFS or OS according to number of LNs involved.
— CONCLUSION:
— No advantage to intensifying cyclophosphamide in adriamycin/cyclophosphamide regimen.

● NSABP-B25.
[DeCillis A, Proc Am Soc Clin Oncol 16:(A459) 1997].
[Oncology News International 7(2 suppl 1): 16, 1998].
— Evaluation of dose intensity and increasing total dose of cyclophosphamide.
— 2548 ♀ with operable, LN(+) breast cancer, randomized.
— Completed accrual 2/94.

Dose intense cyclophosphamide			
	Group I	Group II	Group III
Adriamycin (A)	60 mg/m² q 21 d × 4	60 mg/m² q 21 d × 4	60 mg/m² q 21 d × 4
Cyclophosphamide	1200 mg/m² q 21 d × 4	2400 mg/m² q 21 d × 2	2400 mg/m² q 21 d × 4

— All 3 groups received the same dose of Adriamycin, 60 mg/m² i.v. on day 1 q 3 weeks × 4.

— All ♀ ≥ 50 years old received tamoxifen 10 mg po b.i.d. starting on day 1 of chemotherapy × 5 years.

— RESULTS:
— At 4-year follow-up DFS did not differ across the three treatment groups, ranging from 62% for Group I to 70% for Group 3.
— The 4-year overall survival differed even less, with a range of 80–82%.
— The higher and more intense cyclophosphamide doses were associated with an increased incidence of more severe side effects (leukemia).
— 12 cases of acute leukemia and 4 cases of myelodysplasia have been reported among the 2548 ♀ participants.

— CONCLUSION:
  — This is the second NSABP trial that has failed to show an improvement in DFS or OS with ↑ cyclophosphamide dose and cyclophosphamide dose intensification.

● [Levine M, J Clin Oncol 16: 2651–2658, 1998].
  — 710 pre- or peri-menopausal ♀ with LN(+) breast cancer were Randomized after surgery.
  Group I: CMF q month × 6.
  Cyclophosphamide 100 mg/m^2 p.o. days 1–14.
  Methotrexate 40 mg/m^2 i.v. days 1 and 8.
  Fluorouracil 600 mg/m^2 i.v. days 1 and 8.

  vs.

  Group II. CEF q month × 6.
  Cyclophosphamide 75 mg/m^2 p.o. days 1–14.
  Epirubicin 60 mg/m^2 i.v. days 1 and 8.
  Fluorouracil 500 mg/m^2 i.v. days 1 and 8.
  — ♀ receiving CEF received antibiotic prophylaxis which consisted of Cotrimoxazole (Septra) 2 tablets p.o. b.i.d. for the duration of chemotherapy.
  — If the patient could not tolerate Septra, then Norfloxacin 400 mg p.o. b.i.d. or Ciprofloxacin 500 mg p.o. b.i.d. was used.
  — Colony stimulating factors were not used.

— Median follow-up: 59 months.

— RESULTS:
  — Recurrence:
    — CMF → 169/359 ♀.
    — CEF → 132/359 ♀.
  — 5-year relapse-free survival rates:
    — CMF → 53%.
    — CEF → 63% (P = 0.009).
  — Death
    — CMF → 107 ♀.
    — CEF → 85 ♀.
  — 5-year actuarial survival rates:
    — CMF → 70%.
    — CEF → 77% (P = 0.03).

- Febrile/neutropenia requiring hospitalization.
  - CMF → 1.1%.
  - CEF → 8.5%.
- Congestive heart failure.
  - CMF → 1 ♀.
  - CEF → 0 ♀.
- Acute leukemia.
  - CMF → 0 ♀.
  - CEF → 5 ♀.

- CONCLUSION:
  - Intense CEF regimen proved to be superior to standard CMF regimen in terms of both disease-free survival and overall survival in premenopausal ♀ with axillary LN(+).
  - The high incidence of acute leukemia in the CEF arm needs to be further studied to confirm if it is reproducible.
    - Longterm follow-up of current ongoing Randomized trials in Europe using different doses of epirubicin and cyclophosphamide among premenopausal ♀ with high risk breast cancer will help us determine the answer to this question.

Sequencing of adjuvant chemotherapy and radiation therapy
[Gage I, Current Opinion in Oncology 9(6): 527–531, 1997].

- The international consensus panel at the 1995 conference on Adjuvant Therapy of Primary Breast Cancer concluded that adjuvant radiotherapy could be safely delayed until adjuvant chemotherapy was completed until the conclusions of ongoing studies become available.

- NSABP-B15 and B16.
  [Mamoumas EP, Breast Cancer Res Treat 41: 219(1) 1996].
  - Prospective randomized trials.
  - Did not show an ↑ risk of local recurrence in ♀ with an up to 12 weeks delay in receiving XRT.

- International Breast Cancer Study Group (IBCSG).
  [Wallgren A. Int J Radiat Oncol Biol Phys 35: 649–659, 1996].
  - Two prospective Randomized trials evaluated the surgery-radiation interval.
  - All ♀ had (−) margins of resection.

- Pre-menopausal and peri-menopausal ♀ received CMF × 6, then XRT.

  vs.

- 3 cycles of CMF, then XRT, then there was a subsequent randomization to three more cycles of CMF vs. no more chemotherapy.
- Post-menopausal ♀ received tamoxifen + XRT.

  vs.

- Tamoxifen + CMF × 3, followed by XRT.
- RESULTS:
  - 4-year crude rate.
  - No significant differences in local recurrences were noted among the ♀ in each group.

- [Recht A, New Engl J Med 334: 1356–1361, 1996].
  - 244 ♀ with stage I/II breast cancer found to be at increased risk of having distant metastases.
  - Patients at high risk were defined to have:
    - (+)LN.
    - ER(−).
    - Invasion of lymphatic vessels by tumor.
  - The women were prospectively randomized to receive a 12 week course of chemotherapy before or after radiotherapy, 'upfront-out-back'.
  - All women had breast conserving surgery.

  - The radiation regimen:
    - The entire breast received 45 Gy in 25 fractions with a boost to the primary tumor site of 16–18 Gy. Adjuvant radiotherapy to lymph nodes was left up to the discretion of the radiotherapist.

  - Chemotherapy regimen:
    - Methotrexate 200 mg/m^2 I.V. on days # 1 and # 15.
    - Leucovorin 10 mg/m^2 p.o. q 6 h × 12 doses on days # 2 and # 16.
    - Fluorouracil 500 mg/m^2 i.v. on day # 1.
    - Cyclophosphamide 500 mg/m^2 i.v. on day # 1.
    - Doxorubicin 45 mg/m^2 i.v. on day # 3.
    - Prednisone 40 mg/m^2 p.o. days # 1 through # 5.
    - Cycles were repeated q 21 days × 4 cycles.

- RESULTS:
  - 5-year crude rate.
  - Local recurrence.
    - 5% for XRT upfront.
    - 13% for chemotherapy upfront.
  - Distant failure.
    - 32% for XRT upfront.
    - 20% for chemotherapy upfront.
  - 5-year survival rate without distant recurrence.
    - 64% for XRT upfront.
    - 75% for chemotherapy upfront.
  - $P = 0.05$.

- CONCLUSION:
  - The study suggests that for this high risk group of women, undergoing breast conservation therapy, it is preferable to give a 12 week course of chemotherapy followed by radiation therapy, because it improves both control of distant disease and survival.
    - Provided margins of resection are (−).
    - If margins of resection are (+), or close → re-excise prior to chemotherapy to ↓ risk of ipsilateral breast cancer recurrence.
  - Limitations of the study:
  - Relatively short median follow-up (< 5 years).
  - Too few patients received tamoxifen to allow the evaluation of its effect.

- EORTC.
  [5th EORTC Breast Cancer Working Conference, Leuven, Belgium A 293, 1991].
  - 248 LN(+) ♀, after mastectomy (M), were Randomized to three groups:
    - Group A: M → CMF × 6 → XRT.
    - Group B: M → XRT → CMF × 6.
    - Group C: M → CMF × 3 → XRT → CMF × 3.

- CONCLUSION:
  - At 10 years, local control and DFS were significantly improved among the patients treated in the 'sandwich' arm (Group C).
    - DFS rates were 57% in Group C, 41% in Group B, and 46% in Group A ($P = 0.05$).

Timing of adjuvant chemotherapy

- Ludwig Breast Cancer Study Group.
  [Goldhirsch A, Monogr Natl Cancer Inst 1: 55–70, 1986].
  [LBCSG, New Engl J Med 319: 677–683, 1988].
  − A Randomized prospective trial of LN(+) patients.
  − Designed to determine the optimal timing of post-operative chemotherapy administration.
  − No advantage to the immediate (perioperative) use of chemotherapy compared to the initiation of treatment 4–5 weeks after surgery.
  − The regimen used consisted of cyclophosphamide, methotrexate, fluorouracil, and prednisone (CMFP).

Duration of adjuvant chemotherapy

- The standard duration of chemotherapy is four to six cycles over a period of 3–6 months.

- Milan II:
- [Tancini G, J Clin Oncol 1: 2–10, 1983].
  − Prospective Randomized study.
  − 5-year results:
    − 6 months of CMF as good as 12 months of CMF.

  [Bonadonna G, Cancer Res 52: 2127–2137, 1992].
  − 14-year results:
    − A trend favoring 6 months of CMF was evident.

- Southeastern Cancer Study Group (SEG).
  [SEG, Adjuvant Therapy of Cancer, 5:347, 1987].
  − ♀ with operable breast cancer and (+)LN were randomized.
  − 6 months of CMF as good as 12 months of CMF.

- Ludwig Study:
  [LBCSG, New Engl J Med 319: 677–683, 1988].
  − 1229 LN(+) ♀.
  − 6 months appear to be superior to 1 month of CMF.

- Canadian Study.
  [Levine MN, J Clin Oncol 8: 1217–1225, 1990].
  − Randomized study in ♀ with stage II breast cancer.

— Adjuvant chemotherapy administered for 12 vs. 36 weeks.
— Trial had to be prematurely stopped when a significant DFS and OS
  advantage was discovered in the 36 week chemotherapy group.

● **NSABP-B15.**
  [Fisher B, J Clin Oncol 8(9): 1483–1496, 1990].
  — 2194 ♀ with operable breast cancer.
  — ♀ < 49 years old or 50–59 years old, with PR(−) tumor regardless
    of ER status (tamoxifen non-responsive).
  — LN(+) patients.
  — Patients randomized to three groups after surgery.
  — Compared A.C. (4 doses; ∼ 2 months; 63 days) vs. CMF × 6 months.
    — Group I: Adriamycin 60 mg/m^2 i.v.
                 Cyclophosphamide 600 mg/m^2 i.v.
                 q 21 days × 4 cycles.
    — Group II: AC identical to Group I
                 6 months after last dose of AC received, CMF was
                 begun.
                 Cyclophosphamide 750 mg/m^2 i.v.
                 Methotrexate 40 mg/m^2 i.v. day 1 and 8.
                 Fluorouracil 600 mg/m^2 i.v. day 1 and 8.
                 q 21 days × 3 cycles.

	Group I	Group II		Group III
Adria (A)	60 mg/m^2 i.v.	60 mg/m^2 i.v.		
Cyclo (C)	600 mg/m^2 i.v.	600 mg/m^2 i.v.	750 mg/m^2 i.v.	100 mg/m^2 p.o. days 1–14
Metho (M)			40 mg/m^2 i.v. days 1 and 8	40 mg/m^2 i.v. days 1 and 8
5FU			600 mg/m^2 i.v. days 1 and 8	600 mg/m^2 i.v. days 1 and 8
Timing	q 21 days × 4 cycles	q 21 days × 4 cycles	Starting 6 months after end of AC. Q 21 days × 3 cycles	q 28 days × 6 cycles

- Group III: Conventional CMF.
  Cyclophosphamide 100 mg/m² p.o. day 1-14.
  Methotrexate 40 mg/m² i.v. day 1 and 8.
  Fluorouracil 600 mg/m² i.v. day 1 and 8.
  q 28 days × 6 cycles.

- 13-year follow-up.
  - No significant difference in DFS or OS in the three groups.
  - CONCLUSION:
    - Felt AC (group I) to be better since less toxic.
    - Note, no benefit of re-induction with CMF.

Side effects of chemotherapy
Please refer to the specific section on side effects of chemotherapy in the metastatic breast cancer section, page 138.

Adjuvant tamoxifen in premenopausal ♀

- In most trials with younger ♀, tamoxifen was administered with chemotherapy.

- Overview study [EBCTCG, Lancet 339: 1-15 and 71-85, 1992].
  - Not a clear benefit; in overview only 1% difference in mortality (900 deaths vs. 850 patients on tamoxifen).

  - Controversy:
    - Premenopausal ♀ were kept on tamoxifen less time (mean 1.6 years) than postmenopausal ♀ (mean 2.6 years).
    - Some experts believe tamoxifen offers a greater benefit in premenopausal ♀ than suggested by the overview study.

  - Tamoxifen.
    - Safe (?).
    - More than 2 years is better than less than 2 years.
    - 5 years is the standard of care.
    - ↑ DFS and OS.
    - May benefit bone density in postmenopausal ♀.
      [Love RR, New Engl J Med 326: 852-856, 1992].
      - In premenopausal ♀ bone mineral density was ↓ during the first 2 years of therapy in a British chemoprevention tamoxifen trial.

- May benefit blood lipid levels.
  [Love RR, J Natl Cancer Inst 86: 1534–1539, 1994].
- May ↓ risk of contralateral breast cancer.
  [Rutqvist LE, J Natl Cancer Inst 83: 1299–1306, 1991].

- **NSABP-B14.**
  [Constantino J, Proc Am Soc Clin Onc 12: 64(A59) 1993].
  [Fisher B, J Natl Cancer Inst 88: 1529–1542, 1996].
  - 2843 ♀ with LN(−), ER(+) breast cancers.
  - Randomized to tamoxifen 20 mg/day vs. placebo.
  - 8 years out now showing improved overall survival for tamoxifen group.
  - Positive benefit with tamoxifen in both pre- and postmenopausal ♀.
  - 1989 at time of publication, 77 vs. 83% DFS.
  - At 7 years follow-up, the treated group had 9% improvement in DFS.
  - ↓ incidence of contralateral breast cancer.
  - ↓ disease recurrence and ↑ DFS in pre and postmenopausal women.
  - NSABP-B14 found that tamoxifen provides no benefit beyond 5 years.
  [J Natl Cancer Institute 87: 1829, 1995].

- **Scottish Trial.**
  [Zaire J, Lancet 2: 171–175, 1987].
  - Conducted from 4/78–9/84.
  - Premenopausal LN(+) excluded.
  - 1312 patients; premenopausal LN (−), postmenopausal LN (+) and LN (−).
  - Randomized to adjuvant tamoxifen 20 mg p.o. q.d. × 5 years.
  - RESULTS:
    - Both pre/post-menopausal ♀ had an overall survival advantage from adjuvant tamoxifen.
    - 15% survival advantage at 8 years.

- **Scottish Trial.**
  [Stewart HJ, Br J Cancer 74(2): 297–299, 1996].
  - ♀ in the previous Scottish tamoxifen trial.
  - Re-randomized at the end of 5 years.
    - Stop tamoxifen at 5 years vs. continue tamoxifen indefinitely.
  - Preliminary analysis of 342 ♀ at a median follow-up of 6 years, suggests a significant benefit from continuing tamoxifen beyond 5 years is unlikely.
    - May ↑ risk of endometrial cancer.

- ECOG 5181 and ECOG 4181.
  [Tormey DC, J Natl Cancer Inst 88: 1828–1833, 1996].
  – 194 ♀ with LN(+)/ER(+) breast cancer.
    – 25% of ♀ had ER(−) tumors.
  – Treated with surgery followed by 1 year of chemotherapy and 5 years of tamoxifen.
  – Randomized to two concurrent Eastern Cooperative Oncology Group (ECOG) adjuvant trails.
    – Continuous tamoxifen vs. observation after 5 years of tamoxifen.
  – 107 premenopausal ♀ (ECOG 5181).
  – 87 postmenopausal ♀ (ECOG 4181).
  – Median follow-up 5.6 years since randomization.
  – RESULTS:
    – No statistical significance was noted in either time to relapse or survival between ♀ continuing to receive tamoxifen and those on observation after having received 5 years of tamoxifen. 85 vs. 73%, respectively. $P = 0.01$.

Conclusions of above studies:

- Adjuvant tamoxifen is prescribed for 5 years in LN(−) ♀.
- The optimal duration of therapy in LN(+) ♀ is not known, but is at least 5 years.
- Tamoxifen beyond 5 years remains unsupported by data.

- Long term tamoxifen follow-up.
  – Incidence of endometrial carcinoma is 2/1000 patients per year at 20 mg q.d. in U.S. studies.
    – > 100 cases reported worldwide.
  – There is no clear consensus on how to follow these patients, however, ♀ on tamoxifen should have yearly gynecological examination and be aware of this rare but very serious toxicity.
  – Some experts recommend at baseline and q 6 months to 1 year.
    – Vaginal ultrasound.
    – CA125.
    – Endometrial biopsies.

Adjuvant immunotherapy
[Lacour J, Eur J Surg Oncol 14: 311–316, 1988].
- Most trials with immunotherapy have failed to demonstrate an advantage.

- No current role for immunotherapy.

ADJUVANT CHEMOTHERAPY IN POSTMENOPAUSAL BREAST CANCER

- Six year ECOG Study.
  [Taylor SG, J Clin Oncol 7: 879–889, 1989].
  - 265 postmenopausal, LN(+) ♀.
  - 74 months median follow up.
  - Compared CMFP(prednisone) vs. CMFP + Tamox vs. observe × 1 year.
  - There is some benefit to adjuvant chemotherapy (CMFP ± tamoxifen) in ER (−) ♀ (found in subset analysis).
  - Numbers in trial are very small.

- NSABP-B16.
  [Fisher B, J Clin Oncol 8:1005–1018, 1990].
  - 1124 postmenopausal, HR(+) ♀, > 50 years old.
  - Randomized trial.
  - Tamoxifen vs. Tamoxifen + AC vs. Tamoxifen + Melphalan + 5FU + Adriamycin.
  - Benefit to Tamoxifen + AC arm.
  - All AC given in ∼ 2 months (63 days): four cycles, q 3 weeks with concurrent tamoxifen (continued for 5 years).
  - Recent data indicates a disease free and overall survival advantage for doxorubicin + cyclophosphamide + tamoxifen (ACT) over tamoxifen alone in LN(+) patients, between age 50–59 with PR(+) tumors, and those older than 59, regardless of the steroid receptor content of the cancers.

- In postmenopausal women with LN(+) and ER(+) breast cancer, adjuvant tamoxifen prolongs DFS and OS.

- A National Cancer Institute consensus development conference in 1985 found: no indication for routine chemotherapy for older post-operative patients.

- The overview study (Meta-Analysis II).
  [EBCTCG, Lancet (11 January): 71–85, 1992].
  - Evaluated 30000 women Randomized to tamoxifen.
  - Women on tamoxifen for 2 years did better than those on it for 1 year.
  - Benefit greater in older women (postmenopausal) even if ER(−).

— ER(−) premenopausal women → no benefit from tamoxifen.
— Survival benefit from tamoxifen was greater at 10 years than at 5 years.
— Looked at all the Randomized trials between 1970 and 1985 in North America and Europe.
— The overview confirmed:
  — In patients under the age of 50, receiving CMF or its variant, the odds of relapse are reduced by 1/3rd and the odds of mortality by 1/4th.
  — Although CMF does cause amenorrhea, especially in older pre-meno-pausal women, women who do not become amenorrheic still benefit.
— The overview in postmenopausal women, found that the odds of relapse and death were reduced by 19 and 3%, respectively, neither of which was statistically significant.
— Significant DFS and OS benefit up to age 70, has been reported in the third Meta-Analysis (In press 1998).

● SWOG and ECOG.
  [Dressler LG, Proc Am Soc Clin Oncol 9: 87 (A81), 1990].
  — A trial by the Southwest Oncology Group and the Eastern Cooperative Oncology Group supported the Consensus conclusion above:
  — At 4.3 years median follow-up, no advantage to CMF + vincristine + prednisone + tamoxifen (CMFVPT) over tamoxifen alone was found in postmenopausal patients with ER(+), LN(+) disease.

● Italian Study.
  [Boccardo F, J Clin Oncol 8: 1310–1320, 1990].
  — Multicenter Italian study.
  — LN(+), ER(+) breast cancer patients.
  — Found that tamoxifen was equivalent to chemotherapy + tamoxifen in postmenopausal patients, and both superior to chemotherapy alone.

Side effects of chemotherapy

Please refer to the specific section on side effects of chemotherapy in the metastatic breast cancer section, page 138.

Chemotherapy + Tamoxifen

[Kennedy MJ, Current Opinion in Oncology 9(6): 532–539, 1997]

- NSABP-B09.
  [Fisher B, J Clin Oncol 4: 459–471, 1986].
  – 1858 ♀ (779 premenopausal) randomized to:
    – Chemotherapy alone.
         vs.
    – Chemotherapy plus tamoxifen.
  – Chemotherapy with melphalan and 5-fluorouracil (PF).
  – There was no overall significant benefit observed for tamoxifen in ER(–) patients.
  – Significant improvement in DFS was observed in ER(+) patients that received tamoxifen.
  – Subset analysis showed ♀ 60–70 years of age benefitted from tamoxifen even if the tumor was ER(–).
  – The advantage observed in postmenopausal ♀ did not hold true for premenopausal ♀.
  – Since the completion of this trial, tamoxifen has been found to inhibit cellular uptake of melphalan.

- International Breast Cancer Study Group (IBCSG).
  [IBCSG, J Clin Oncol 15: 1385–1394, 1997].
  – 1266 post-menopausal ♀ with LN(+) breast cancer.
  – Randomized to tamoxifen alone × 5 years
         vs.
  – Tamoxifen and three or six cycles of CMF.
  – RESULTS:
    – 5-year disease-free survival rates.
      – 64% for ♀ receiving tamoxifen + CMF.
      – 57% for ♀ receiving tamoxifen alone.

- NSABP-B20.
  [Fisher B, J Natl Cancer Inst 89(22): 1652–1654, 1997].
  – 2306 ♀ with LN(–), ER(+) breast cancer after surgery were randomized:
    771 ♀→tamoxifen alone.
    767 ♀→methotrexate, fluorouracil, and tamoxifen (MFT).
    768 ♀→cyclophosphamide, methotrexate, fluorouracil, tamoxifen (CMFT).

  – Five years of follow-up.

- RESULTS:
  - Chemotherapy plus tamoxifen resulted in significantly better DFS than tamoxifen alone ($P < 0.01$).
    - 90% DFS for MFT.
    - 89% DFS for CMFT.
    - 85% DFS for tamoxifen alone.
  - MFT and CMFT compared to tamoxifen alone ↓ risk of ipsilateral breast cancer after lumpectomy.
  - Chemotherapy and tamoxifen resulted in a better DFS than tamoxifen alone.
  - Survival benefit found in MFT and CMFT when compared to tamoxifen alone.
    - 97% survival for MFT.
    - 96% survival for CMFT.
    - 94% survival for tamoxifen alone.
  - No subgroup of patients evaluated in this study failed to benefit from chemotherapy.

- SWOG 8814, Intergroup Study (INT) 0100.
  [Albain K, Proc Am Soc Clin Oncol 16: 128].
  - 1550 ♀ with LN(+)/ER(+) breast cancer.
  - Randomized to tamoxifen alone
    vs.
  - CAF with concurrent or sequential tamoxifen.
  - RESULTS:
    - 4-year estimated DFS was superior for the combined chemo/hormonal therapy vs. tamoxifen alone.
    - 79 vs. 72%, $P = 0.001$.
    - No difference noted in overall survival.

- [Pritchard KI, J Clin Oncol 14: 2731–2737, 1996].
  [Pritchard KI, Proc Am Soc Clin Oncol 13: 65(A61), 1994].
  - National Cancer Institute of Canada Clinical Trials Group Breast Cancer Site Group.
  - 705 Postmenopausal ♀, ER/PR(+), LN(+).
  - Randomized:
    - Group I: CMF + Tamoxifen (30 mg/day × 2 years).
    Group II: Tamoxifen alone (30 mg/day × 2 years).

— Thrombotic events, including pulmonary emboli, were significantly increased in
Group I.
  — 13.6% (48 of 353 patients).
                    vs.
— Group II.
  — 2.6% (5 of 352 patients). $P < 0.0001$.

LOCAL BREAST RECURRENCE

- Local recurrence is demoralizing.

- Thought to be a marker of poor prognosis.

- At the time of local recurrence, the patient should be completely restaged.

- In ♀ s/p mastectomy:
  - ~ 80–90% of local recurrences occur within the first 5 years after mastectomy.
  - Recent data suggest that in ♀ s/p chemotherapy, 40% of local recurrences occur after 5 years.

  - ~ 25–30% of local recurrences have preceding distant metastases.

  - ~ 25% of ♀ are diagnosed as having concurrent local recurrence and distant metastases.

  - Virtually all ♀ with chest wall recurrence develop metastatic disease.

- In ♀ s/p breast conserving therapy:
  - ~ 10% of ♀ have simultaneous local breast recurrence in distant metastases.

  - In the prospective Randomized trials conducted, 10-year local recurrence rates range from 4–20% with breast-conserving therapy and XRT.
  - Recurrences begin to appear ~ 2–3 years after treatment.
  - And continue to appear at the rate of 1–2% per year.

  - Breast recurrence after breast conserving therapy is not associated with ↑ risk of distant recurrence.

- There is a persistent risk of local recurrence through 20 years of follow-up, noted in a nonrandomized study. [Kurtz JM, Cancer 63: 1912–1917, 1989].
  - This study evaluated 1593 ♀ with stage I and stage II breast cancer who were treated with breast conserving therapy.

- There are 2 major types of local recurrence:

  - The most common one is a solitary recurrence at the site of the original tumor.
    - Has not been shown to influence overall survival.
    - Prognosis is good.
    - Salvage mastectomy is indicated for recurrence in the breast status post lumpectomy and XRT.

  - The second type is more diffuse, sometimes disseminated throughout the breast (carcinoma-en-cuirasse).
    - May involve skin and dermal lymphatics.
    - Nodules and ulceration are often present.
    - May act as distant metastatic disease.
    - Poor prognosis.
    - Very resistant to treatment.
    - Often requires aggressive chemotherapy prior to palliative mastectomy.
    - Autogenous tissue is better than tissue expansion for immediate reconstruction in previously irradiated breasts.

- Risk factors for recurrence after breast conservation therapy.
  [Fourquet A, Int J Radiat Oncol Biol Phys 17: 719–725, 1989].

  1. Residual malignant calcifications on mammogram.

  2. Residual tumor (+ margins)
      [Schnitt SJ, Cancer 74: 1746–1751, 1994].

  3. EIC with (+) margins.
      [Schnitt SJ, Cancer 74: 1746–1751, 1994].

  4. (+) Lymphatic vessel invasion.
      [Veronesi U, J Natl Cancer Inst 87: 19–27, 1995].

  5. (+) vascular invasion.

  6. High proliferative rate.

  7. Age < 40 (young age).
      [Borger J, J Clin Oncol 12: 653–660, 1994].

— Netherlands Cancer Institute.
— Retrospective review of 1026 stage I/II breast cancer patients.
— Treated with breast conservation (local excision (1–2 cm margins) with axillary LN dissection followed by XRT).
— Actuarial local recurrence 4% at 5 years.
— Median follow-up 66 months.
— Used more extensive breast resection (compared to lumpectomy) and higher doses of XRT (65–75 Gy) compared to most American studies.

— CONCLUSIONS:
  — Young age and (+) vascular invasion are independent predictive factors for local recurrence.
  — Women < 40 years old had 8% local recurrence at 5 years.
  — Tumors with (+) vascular invasion had 11% local recurrence at 5 years.
— Limitation of study [Harris JR, J Clin Oncol 12: 647–649, 1994].
  — The small number of ♀ with local recurrence, 38 as the first site of failure, and a total of 45, limits the statistical power to identify risk factors.

— Tumor size, nodal status, histologic grade and HR status do not seem to be associated with ↑ risk of local recurrence, on multivariate analysis.

● In other studies T_2 tumors, with (+) or narrow margins, and (+) LN, without adjuvant systemic therapy have also been reported as being risk factors for local recurrence.

Treatment modalities after mastectomy

- Hyperthermia.

  [Kapp DS, Int J Radiat Oncol Biol Phys 35: 1117–1121, 1996].

  [Amichetti M, Am J Clin Oncol 14: 60–65, 1991].

  [Scott R, Int J Radiat Oncol Biol Phys 15: 711–716, 1988].

  – In previously non-irradiated patients who had a local recurrence after mastectomy excellent results have been achieved in some studies combining hyperthermia with XRT.

  – Hyperthermia is used in patients who have generally been previously treated with radiation, therefore these patients are at a higher risk of developing radiation-induced complications.

  [Vernon CC, Int J Radiat Oncol Biol Phys 35(4):731–744, 1996].

  – Combined results from five Randomized trials between 1988 and 1991.

  – 306 ♀ with superficial localized breast cancer were randomized to: XRT ± hyperthermia.

  – Overall CR for XRT alone → 41%.

  – Overall CR for XRT + hyperthermia → 59%.

  – RESULTS:

    – The greatest benefit was observed in ♀ with recurrent lesions in previously irradiated areas, where further XRT was limited to low doses.

  – CONCLUSION:

    – The results of the five Randomized trials combined has demonstrated the efficacy of hyperthermia as an adjunct to XRT in the treatment of recurrent breast cancer, particularly in the previously irradiated chest wall.

  [Bornstein BA, Int J Radiat Oncol Biol Phys 25: 79–85, 1992].

  – Other studies have found no benefit in adding hyperthermia to XRT.

  – Therefore its use remains controversial.

  – Hyperthermia may ↑ risk of XRT complications, especially among previously irradiated patients.

- Interferon-B.

  [Gundersen S, Eur J Cancer 27: 220–221, 1991].

  – Intralesional interferon-B, given simultaneously with external beam radiation resulted in four CR's in previously irradiated patients.

- Topical treatment.
  [Elkort RJ, Cancer 46: 647–653, 1980].
  — Topical treatments may be of great relief in controlling local infection and pain.
    — 0.5% silver nitrate soaked dressings along with local debridement can be very helpful.

CHARGES RELATED TO BREAST CANCER TREATMENT IN EUROPE

Tumorectomy (lumpectomy)	$1400–1800
Segmentectomy + axillary dissection	$1500–2000
Quandrantectomy	$1500–2500
Mastectomy	$2000–3000
Primary unilateral breast reconstruction free flap	$4000–8500
Primary unilateral breast reconstruction implant*	$6500–8500
Secondary unilateral breast reconstruction free flap	$8500–10 000
Secondary unilateral breast reconstruction implant	$5000–7000
Primary bilateral breast reconstruction free flap	$10 000–13 000
Primary bilateral breast reconstruction implant	$7500–9500
Secondary bilateral breast reconstruction free flap	$10 000–13 000
Secondary bilateral breast reconstruction implant	$7000–9000

Chemotherapy: (anti-emetic and growth factors included)
    CMF × 6
    CAF × 6
	$5400–6100
	$6000–6500

Radiotherapy	$2500–3000
Tamoxifen (Nolvadex) × 5 years	$1500

* In this list, the costs for surgical revisions after implant reconstruction are not included. As those revisions can be frequent, especially following radiotherapy, the long-term costs for implants will be higher than breast reconstruction with autologous tissue.

METASTATIC BREAST CANCER

- Metastases occur prior to the initial treatment in most patients; otherwise, surgery would cure breast cancer.

- The majority of deaths are caused by the growth of metastases.

- [Clark, GM, J Clin Oncol 5: 55–61, 1987].
  ♀ with metastatic breast cancer have a median survival rate of ~2 years.

- Breast cancer spreads via:
  – Direct infiltration into the breast parenchyma.
  – Via tumor emboli to lymphatics.
  – Along mammary ducts.
  – Hematogeneously to distant metastases.

- One-third to one-half of all patients with primary invasive breast cancer will eventually develop disseminated disease.

- Relapses occur at an approximately constant rate in approximately the first 10 years, then continue at a progressively slower rate indefinitely.

- Can recur up to 30 years later [Rutqvist LE, Cancer 55: 658–665, 1985].

- Bone is the most common site of first distant relapse in all reported series. The next most common sites are lung (~20%) and pleura (~8%).

- Solitary first relapses to the liver are relatively rare (~5%), although liver involvement is documented in more than 1/2 of cases at autopsy.

- CNS metastases as a first site of relapse are also rare (~4% of the cases).

- Not curable; goal is palliation.

- Categories:
  – Loco-regional disease.
  – Bone only.
  – Visceral disease.
  – Visceral crises.

Loco-regional disease
Chest wall recurrence

- If > 4 $(+)$LN then chance of chest wall recurrence is 20–50% in lifetime, if not irradiated.
  - If XRT up-front.
    - 90% success in local control.
    - 10% still recur locally.
  - If XRT is given when local recurrence develops then 50% chance of local control.

- Adjuvant post-mastectomy XRT.
  [Cuzick J, J Clin Oncol 12(3): 447–453, 1994].
  - Markedly decreases local relapse rate and may improve survival.

- Radiotherapy to chest wall after mastectomy has been reported to decrease the probability of response to subsequent chemotherapy. However, this relationship has never been found for breast irradiated after breast conserving surgery.

- Treatment:
  - It is difficult to control gross disease by XRT alone.
  - Thus, for an isolated chest wall or axillary recurrence.
    - Resect if possible.
  - However, these patients frequently recur with multiple nodules which are unresectable, or if technically resectable often rapidly develop recurrences elsewhere after resection.
  - Local XRT markedly reduces the risk of loco-regional failure.
  - Following resection, local XRT is usually directed at the recurrent site, chest wall and supraclavicular area.
  - Most patients with a loco-regional failure will eventually manifest distant metastases and therefore the situation is essentially palliative. Nevertheless, some of these patients do live a long time.
    - Therefore aggressive/comprehensive treatment of the loco-regional site is necessary.
    - Uncontrolled extensive loco-regional disease has a very negative impact on patient's quality of life.
  - ER/PR$(+)$ tumors may respond well to tamoxifen in previously irradiated ♀.

- Risks of treatment.
  - There appears to be a slight increase in cardiac events following loco-regional XRT in patients with left sided lesions. Risk is reduced by careful treatment planning.

- Intraarterial cytotoxic therapy (CONTROVERSIAL).
  [Stephens FO, Cancer 66(4): 645–650, 1990].
  - May be beneficial for carcinoma en cuirasse.
  - Increased concentrations of cytotoxic agents can be delivered locally and with longer infusion times.
    [Koyama H, Cancer 36: 1603–1612, 1975].
  - Infusion may be via the internal mammary, lateral thoracic or by subclavian artery.
  - True benefit is not known.
  - There are no current randomized trials.

Brachial plexopathy
[Kori SH, Oncology 9(8): 756–760, 1995].

- In cancer patients the most common causes of brachial plexopathy are metastatic spread of tumor and radiation injury.
  - To distinguish between these two entities is not always easy.

- Radiation Injury.
  [Pierce SM, Int J Radiat Oncol Biol Phys 23: 915–923, 1992].
  - Incidence.
    - ~ 1–1.8% of patients.
  - Predisposing factors:
    - Radiation dose.
      - ↑ incidence when axillary dose of radiation is > 50 Gy.
    - Treatment technique.
      - Three field technique has higher incidence than two field technique.
    - Concomitant or previous chemotherapy.
  - Onset of symptoms.
    - ~ 7.5 months to 6 years after the radiation is completed.

  - Clinical features.
    - Numbness.
    - Paresthesias/dysesthesia.

— Swelling.
— Weakness of arm.
— <u>Pain</u> and Horner's syndrome are not part of the typical presentation, in contrast to brachial plexus injury due to metastases.
— Diagnostic studies.
  — Plain films, tomograms and bone scans are not useful.
  — MRI is better than CT.
  — Electromyographic studies can be very useful.

— Prognosis and treatment.
  — ∼ 80% of patients improved spontaneously or 20% had progressive deterioration.
  — Instituting physical therapy early helps prevent lymphedema, frozen shoulder, posture induced muscle spasm and muscle atrophy.
  — Tricyclics and anticonvulsants can help control neuropathic pain.
  — Transdermal electrical nerve stimulation (TENS) may be useful for patients with intractable pain.

● Metastatic brachial plexopathy.
  [Harper CM, Neurology 39: 502–506, 1989].
  — Tumors that commonly involve the brachial plexus are from the lung, breast and lymphoma.
  — Onset of symptoms:
    — ∼ 3 months to 14 years.

  — Clinical features.
    — Pain is the most common presenting symptom.
      — Typically the pain begins in the shoulder girdle and radiates to the elbow, medial side of the forearm and the 4th and 5th fingers.
      — Movement of the shoulder ↑ the pain.
      — In some patients pain is localized to the posterior part of the arm or the elbow.
      — Horner's syndrome is a common finding.
        — An MRI of the spine or myelogram to rule out epidural metastases, should be done even if no other signs of cord compression are present.

  — Prognosis and treatment.
    — Prognosis is usually poor.

- Radiation therapy to the plexus with or without chemotherapy can provide pain relief.
- Paravertebral nerve blocks can be very helpful in patients with 1–2 nerve roots involved.
- Dorsal rhizotomy and cordotomy can be tried in patients with intractable pain.
- Tricyclics, anticonvulsants and non-steroidal anti-inflammatory agents and steroids can be helpful.
- Physical therapy and TENS can also be helpful.

Bone only
[Hortobagyi GN, Diseases of the Breast Updates 1(3): 1–11, 1997].

- ♀ with bone only disease frequently have indolent disease and can survive, on average, 4 years with therapy.

- Is the most common site of metastatic spread.
  - 30–40% of all first metastases.
  - More common in the axial skeleton than in the extremities.

  - Complications of bone metastases:
  - Pain.
  - Fractures.
  - Hypercalcemia.

- 40% destruction of bone is necessary before lytic lesion is revealed by plain X-ray.

- Bone scan is good for diagnosis but not for following disease, because bone scan picks up blastic disease. When a lytic lesion heals, it leaves a blastic lesion, so there are lots of false positives.

- The standard treatment for bone metastases is systemic therapy (hormonal and/or cytotoxic).

- Once started tamoxifen or chemotherapy, one can see an ↑ in alkaline phosphatase for 1–2 months, presumably secondary to bone turnover, but then it decreases.

- Endocrine therapy achieves objective tumor response in 25–45% of patients.

- Chemotherapy.
  [Hortobagyi GN, New Engl J Med 335: 1785–1791, 1996].
  — Achieved pain reduction in ~ 30% of patients.
  — ~ 18% of patients showed radiological response.

- Palliative XRT is the standard treatment for pain control if pain persists after hormonal therapy and/or chemotherapy, or in cases of impending fracture in weight bearing areas or spine metastases which may progress to cord compression.
  — Bone pain is relieved by radiotherapy in over 90% of cases.
    — Complete bone pain relief occurs in ~ 30–50%.
  — Three-fourths of treated patients will have evidence of bone healing on X-rays within 3 months.
    — Not a reproducible finding.
  — Few patients develop pathologic fractures after successful radiotherapy.
    — Persistent pain or advancing disease after radiotherapy may indicate the need for surgical fixation.
    — Indications for prophylactic fixation:
      — Cortical bone destruction ≥ 50%.
      — 2.5 cm lesion in the proximal femur.
      — Pathologic avulsion fracture of the lesser trochanter.
      — Persistent stress pain despite irradiation.

- Antiosteolytic biphosphonates.
  — The most commonly used biphosphonates are:
    — Pamidronate 90 mg i.v. over 2–3 h q month.
    — Clodronate 1600 mg p.o. b.i.d.

  — Oral biphosphonates thus far have been associated with:
    — Poor bioavailability (~ 1%).
    — Esophageal irritation.

  — Etidronate is not appropriate for the treatment of bone metastases.

  — Potent inhibitors of osteoclastic bone resorption.

  — Useful in reducing pain, analgesic use, fractures and hypercalcemia.

  — Useful in improving quality of life.

[Hortobagyi GN, New Engl J Med 335: 1785–1791, 1996].
[Hortobagyi GN, J Clin Onc 16(6): 2038–2044, 1998].
- Double-blind Randomized, multi-center, parallel-group trial.
- 382 ♀ with metastatic breast cancer and lytic bone lesions who received chemotherapy, were Randomized.
   Pamidronate 90 mg i.v. in 2-h infusion q 3–4 weeks × 24 months + chemotherapy.
   vs.
   Chemotherapy alone (no Pamidronate).
- The Pamidronate arm found:
   - Delayed onset of first skeletal metastases (13.9 vs. 7 months).
   - ($P < 0.001$).
   - Higher radiological response (34 vs. 19%) ($P = 0.002$).
   - Requirements for palliative XRT were ↓ (33 vs. 19%).
   - Requirements for palliative bone surgery were ↓ (10 vs. 4%).
   - There was no survival difference.
[Conte PF, J Clin Oncol 14: 2552–2559, 1996].
- ♀ with metastatic breast cancer to bone Randomized to:
   - chemotherapy with Pamidronate 45 mg i.v. q 3 weeks.
   vs.
   - chemotherapy alone.
- RESULTS:
   - Time to progression was ↑ by almost 50% in ♀ treated with the biphosphonate (249 days vs. 168 days, $P = 0.02$).

[Diel IJ, N Engl J Med 339: 357–363, 1998]
- 302 ♀ with primary breast cancer and tumor cells in the bone marrow were studied.
- All ♀ underwent standard surgery, followed by standard chemotherapy and/or hormonal therapy.
- ♀ were Randomized to:
   - Group I. 157 ♀ Clodronate 1600 mg p.o. q.d. × 2 years.
      vs.
   - Group II. 145 ♀ standard follow-up (no Clodronate).
- Median follow-up → 36 months.

- RESULTS:
   - Distant metastases
      - 21 ♀ in Clodronate group
         vs.
         42 ♀ in control group ($P < 0.001$).

- Incidence of both bony and visceral metastases was significantly lower in the Clodronate group.
- Death
- 6 ♀ died in Clodronate group
  vs.
  22 ♀ died in the control group.

- Radioactive bone-seeking agents (systemic radiation therapy). [Ben-Josef E, Ann Med 29(1): 31–35, 1997].
  - Strontium-89 and samarium-153.
    - Studies are limited by the small number of patients to date.
    - β-emitters.
    - Have a greater uptake in metastatic bone than in normal bone.
    - Pain relief is achieved in $\sim 80\%$ of the patients for a mean of 8 weeks.
    - Indications:
      - Progressive bone disease after conventional therapy has failed.
    - SIDE EFFECTS: myelosuppression is the dose limiting toxicity.

- Hypercalcemia.
  - Most common metabolic complication of breast cancer.
  - Patients with bone and liver metastases are especially prone to hypercalcemia.
  - Can present with bone pain during tumor flare reactions due to hormonal manipulations.
  - Clinical presentation:
    - Fatigue.
    - Nausea.
    - Constipation.
    - Polyuria.
    - Dehydration.
    - Confusion and somnolence.
  - Treatment:
    - One must decide whether the patient can be managed as an inpatient or as an outpatient.
    - i.v. fluids.
      - Used alone are not sufficient to reduce the calcium to normal levels but are necessary to rehydrate the patient.
    - Steroids.
      - Best for tumor flare associated hypercalcemia.

— For rapid/emergency ↓ in calcium:
— Calcitonin.
   — 8 I.U./Kg intramuscular q 6–8 h × 4 doses.
   — Can be given regardless of volume status or renal function.
— In addition to calcitonin, pamidronate or gallium nitrate is recommended once the patient is rehydrated.
   — Gallium nitrate dose: 350 mg continuous infusion × 3–5 days.
   — Pamidronate dose: 60–90 mg i.v. over 2–3 h.

Visceral disease
[Harris JR, Diseases of the Breast, 1996].

Lung disease
[Kamby C, Cancer 62: 2226–2233, 1988].

• A solitary pulmonary nodule represents a primary lung cancer in more than 50% of patients with breast cancer.

• The lung is the first site of recurrence in 15–25% of patients with metastatic breast cancer.

• The treatment of lung metastases is systemic therapy (hormonal or cytotoxic).
   — If a solitary nodule is resected, systemic therapy should follow.

• Diagnosis:
   — Complete chest CT with special attention to liver and adrenals.
   — Cytologic evaluation from sputum, bronchoscopic washing, or CT guided transthoracic needle biopsy.
   — If these procedures do not yield a diagnosis, video-assisted thoracoscopic surgery can be of great help.
      — Minimally invasive.
      — Definitive tissue is obtained.
      — Direct evaluation of the pleura, ipsilateral peritracheal, and internal mammary lymph nodes.

• Treatment:
[Lanza LA, Ann Thorac Surg 54: 244–247, 1992].
   — Resection of a solitary nodule may be beneficial.
   — Retrospective study.

— Reviewed 37 cases of surgically resected solitary nodules in breast cancer patients and found 49.5% actuarial 5 year survival rate.

Malignant effusions
[Sahn SA, Ann Intern Med 108: 345–349, 1988].
- Pleural effusions.
  — Occur because of pleural metastases.
  — Breast cancer is the most common cause of malignant pleural effusion in ♀.
  — Can be ipsilateral, contralateral, and bilateral.
  — Median survival of patients is 1–2 years.
  — Clinical presentations:
    — Shortness of breath.
    — Cough.
    — Pain.

  — Classically the effusion is an exudate.
    — High protein level (> 3 g/dl).
    — Glucose level is ↓.
    — pH can be normal or low (< 7.3).
      — Patients with a low effusion pH have a shorter median survival. (3.5 months vs. 16.6 months in patients with normal pH).
  — Treatment:
    — Systemic chemotherapy or hormonal manipulations may result in good responses.
    — Local treatment:
      — Intermittent drainage (thoracentesis).
      — Chest tube placement and sclerosis.
        — Drugs used as sclerosing agents:
          — Tetracycline, in USA not available in desired form.
          — Doxycycline is used in its place.
          — Nitrogen mustard.
          — Bleomycin.
      — Thoracoscopy with talc insufflation.

- Pericardial effusions.
  — Occur in breast cancer patients because of tumor involvement or radiation pericarditis.
  — Pericardial involvement by breast cancer is present in ∼ 25% of patients with metastatic disease, by the time of death.

— Responsible for death in < 5% of patients.
— Can lead to cardiac tamponade.

— Symptoms of cardiac tamponade:
  — Dyspnea on exertion.
    — Patient is comfortable at rest.
    — Arterial blood gas at rest shows normal oxygenation.
  — Orthopnea.
  — Chest pain.

— Signs of cardiac tamponade:
  — Tachycardia.
  — Distant heart sounds.
  — ↓ or absent cardiac impulse.
  — Jugular venous distension.
  — Paradoxical movement of the jugular venous pulse.
  — Hypotension and peripheral vascular constriction.

— Diagnoses:
  — Echocardiogram.
    — Mainstay of diagnosis.
  — CT scan.
    — Can be useful, but does not provide physiologic information.

— Local treatment:
  — Pericardial tamponade is a medical emergency and can result in sudden death.
  — Options:
    — Percutaneous pericardial catheter drainage.
    — Subxyphoid pericardial window.
      — Most common treatment.
    — Video-assisted thoracoscopic surgery.
    — Thoracotomy pericardial stripping.
— Systemic therapy:
  — Please refer to the Endocrine and Chemotherapy sections below.

Ocular metastases
[Ratanatharathorn V, Cancer Treat Rev 18: 261–276, 1991].

● Breast cancer is the most common cause of intraocular metastasis in adult females.

- Breast cancer is also the most common tumor to metastasize to the eyelids.

- Simultaneous involvement of the eye and the central nervous system is common.
  - CT/MRI should be performed to rule out CNS metastases.

- Median time from diagnosis of breast cancer to development of ocular metastases is 3–4 years.

- Clinical presentation:
  - For choroid metastases:
    - ↓ visual acuity.
    - Pain.
    - Headache.
    - Photophobia.
  - For metastases to soft tissues of the orbit:
    - Proptosis.
    - Ptosis.
    - Pain.
    - Diplopia.
    - Clinical evidence of a mass.

- Diagnostic imaging:
  - For choroid metastases:
    - Indirect funduscopic examination is the most important test.
    - Ultrasound can help distinguish from melanoma.
    - Fluorescein angiograms may be helpful in differentiating benign from malignant processes.
  - For metastases to soft tissues of the orbit:
    - CT/MRI is essential in the work-up.

- Treatment:
  - Must make sure there are no brain metastases or bilateral ocular disease.
  - Most ocular metastases respond to external-beam XRT.

- Prognosis:
  - Median survival for patients with choroid metastases is 314 days.
  - Median survival for patients with orbital metastases is 794 days.

Brain metastases
[Harris JR, Diseases of the Breast, 1996].

- Overall incidence ranges from 6 to 30%.
  - More likely to affect premenopausal ♀.
  - ER(−) tumors more commonly metastasize to the brain.
  - May occur as a single lesion, multiple lesions, or bilaterally, resulting in cerebral edema, causing a spectrum of manifestations.
    - Up to 50% of cerebral metastases occur as single lesions.
  - Usually not hemorrhagic.
  - Must differentiate from meningioma which occurs at ↑ frequency in this population.
  - < 10% of all patients are alive at 1 year.
  - Clinical presentation:
    - Headache.
      - Most common presentation.
      - Progressive in nature.
      - Papilledema is not common.
        - 25–40% of patients.
    - Mental status changes.
    - Hemiparesis.
    - Focal and neurologic deficits.
      - In ∼ 20% of patients.
    - Gait disturbances.
    - Seizure.
      - Most metastases occur at the junction of the gray and white matter.
      - Occurs in 20–30% of patients with brain metastases.
    - Speech disturbance.

- Diagnostic imaging.
  - CT with contrast and/or MRI with gadolinium enhancement are currently the standard.

- Treatment.
  - Must individualize each case and must take into account: performance status, overall tumor burden, projected survival, and most of all, patient's preference.
  - Symptoms:
    - Steroids.
      - Dexamethasone (Decadron) 4 mg q 6 h.
      - With antacid coverage.

— Anticonvulsants.
  — Reserved only for patients who have already had a seizure.
  — Dilantin.
    — Loading dose: 15 mg/kg.
    — Maintenance: 300–400 mg p.o. qd.
    — ↑ risk of developing Stevens-Johnson syndrome with concurrent XRT.
  — Phenobarbital.
    — Drug of choice if patient is currently undergoing radiation.
    — Loading dose: 120 mg.
    — Maintenance: 30 mg p.o. t.i.d.

— Single brain metastasis:
  [Patchell RA, New Engl J Med 322: 494–500, 1990].
— Recent study showed: surgery, if accessible, followed by whole brain irradiation is superior to radiation alone.
  — Only three patients in the study had breast cancer.
  — Disease should be confined solely to the CNS.
  — Complications of surgery.
    — Permanent neurologic damage.

— Multiple brain metastases.
— Whole brain irradiation is treatment of choice.
  — ~ 4000–4500 cGy over 4 weeks is the recommended treatment.
    — There exists a wide range of accepted dose/fractionation schemes.
  — Retreatment with radiation is possible if symptoms recur.
  — Complications of radiation if patients survive > 1 year.
    — Focal radiation necrosis.
    — Leukoencephalopathy.

— Chemotherapy.
— Agents such as cyclophosphamide, 5FU, platinum, bleomycin, carmustine have been shown to enter brain tumors.
  — Objective responses have been demonstrated with chemotherapy. [Cocconi G, Cancer Invest 8: 327–334, 1990].
  — Cisplatin and etoposide q 3 weeks has been shown to be a highly effective combination in treating brain metastases.
  — [Madajewicz S, Cancer 47: 653–657, 1981] CMF and CAF have also been shown to be useful combinations in the treatment of brain metastases.

— Hormonal therapy.
— Proven useful in a few ER(+) patients.

Epidural metastases
[Harris JR, Diseases of the Breast, 1996].
[Hill ME, Br J Cancer 68: 969–973, 1993].

— Spinal cord compression (SCC) is a true emergency.
— The physician should have a high level of suspicion because the functional outcome of the patient is dependent on the degree of impairment she has whenever the treatment begins.
— Vertebral metastases occur in up to 60% of patients with breast cancer.
— They occur most commonly in the thoracic spine.

- Clinical presentation:
  — Pain.
    — Initial symptom in 96% of patients.
    — Precedes other symptoms by a median of 7 weeks.
    — Often the pain is made worse when the patient is lying on her back and it is relieved when sitting up.
    — Patients often need to sleep sitting up.
    — Valsalva maneuvers and stretching maneuvers make the pain worse.

  — On physical exam, commonly there is tenderness on percussion over the site of the lesion.

  — Myelopathy.
    — Characteristic of spinal cord compression.
    — Includes limb weakness, numbness, paresthesias.
    — Sphincter disturbance.
      — Urinary retention.
      — Urinary urgency.
      — Urge incontinence.
      — Constipation.
    — On physical examination, ↑ tone, ↑ clonus, hyperreflexia, Babinski, distended bladder, and a sensory level may be found.

  — There may be multiple sites of epidural disease.
  — Herpes zoster.

- Diagnostic imaging:
  - For back pain alone, begin with plain films.
  - If high suspicion of SCC, can go straight to MRI.
  - If MRI is (+), the entire spine should be imaged.

- Treatment:
  - Steroids.
    - For suspicion of SCC, before the imaging study, steroids are given.
    - For SCC: 100 mg i.v. of dexamethasone with a slow taper over 2–3 weeks, is given while definitive therapy is being given.
    - For radiculopathy: the steroid doses are lower.

  - XRT.
    - Initial therapy for most patients with SCC.
    - Dose: 3000 cGy in 2 weeks–4500 cGy in 4 weeks.
    - Done on an emergency basis.

  - Surgery.
    - Reserved for:
      - Patients that progress through or relapse after XRT.
      - Patients with unstable spines.
      - Patients with spinal cord compression mostly due to bony fragments in epidural space.
      - Patients lacking definite diagnosis.
    - Some studies have shown better prognosis for ambulation for paraplegic patients receiving vertebral body resection.

  - Chemotherapy.
    - Does not play a significant role.

- Prognosis:
  - The mean survival of breast cancer patients who develop SCC is 5–14 months.
  - Post treatment ambulatory status is the most important factor influencing survival among these patients.

Visceral crises
[Disease of the Breast, 1996].

Lymphangitic spread
[Lower EE, Chest 102: 1113–1117, 1992].
● Clinical presentation:
  — Onset can be insidious or rapid.
  — Progressive dyspnea with minimal exertion.
  — Non-productive cough.
  — Hypoxemia.
  — Fever.
  — Weight loss.
  — Cyanosis.
  — Pleuritic chest pain.
  — Tachypnea.
  — Tachycardia and right heart failure.

● Diagnostic testing:
  — Chest X-ray.
    — Characteristically there is a diffuse reticulonodular pattern that more commonly is bilateral.
    — Pleural effusions have been reported in up to 63% of patients.
    — Hilar and mediastinal lymphadenopathy have also been reported.
    — Up to 40% of patients have a normal chest X-ray.
  — High-resolution CT scan.
    — More sensitive.
    — Beaded thickening of the bronchovascular bundles is thought to be a specific finding.
      — Sarcoidosis is the only other condition in which this radiologic sign has been reported.
  — Pulmonary function tests.
    — Characteristically there is a restrictive pattern with ↓ vital capacity, ↓ total lung capacity and ↓ DLCO (diffusion capacity of carbon dioxide).
    — ABG reveals hypoxemia.
  — When tissue diagnosis is required, bronchoscopy is the procedure of choice.

● Prognosis:
  — Median survival is 5.5–13.5 months.

● Treatment:
  — Chemotherapy is generally recommended.
  — Hormonal therapy may be appropriate for some patients.

Leptomeningeal disease

- In clinical series, the incidence is 2–5%.

- Incidence of leptomeningeal disease is ↑ probably due to patients living longer with breast cancer.

- Incidence in MD Anderson series of 710 patients → 5% at autopsy.

- [Funa K, Br J Cancer 50: 231–233, 1984].
  — Occurs more frequently with lobular carcinoma.

- Natural history → progressive neurological dysfunction, death 4–6 weeks.

- Has been reported in patients without systemic disease.

- Cerebral symptoms often result from hydrocephalus.

- Autopsy series:
  — ~ 8/19 patients with hydrocephalus.
  — Diffuse fibrotic thickening of leptomeninges.
  — Concentration of tumor cells around blood vessels and nerves.

- Clinical presentation:
  — Simultaneous development of multifocal abnormalities at more than one level of the neuraxis.
    — Cranial nerves.
    — Cerebral.
    — Spinal.
  — Cranial nerve involvement.
    — Cranial nerves III, VI, VII most commonly involved.
    — Most commonly experienced symptom is diplopia.
    — Facial weakness and ↓ hearing also occur with frequency.
  — Cerebral involvement.
    — Cerebral symptoms result from obstruction to CSF flow.
      — Headache.
      — Lethargy, confusion, memory loss.
      — Nausea/vomiting.
      — Imbalanced walking.

- Spinal root involvement.
  - Spinal symptoms are the most common presentation.
  - Lower extremity limb weakness along with pain in the spine or limbs.
  - Neck pain, nuchal rigidity (rare).
  - Severe nerve pain anywhere without explanation in a breast cancer patient requires lumbar puncture.

- Cytology is the gold standard for diagnosis.
  [Wasserstrom WR, Cancer 49: 759–772, 1982].
  (+) cytology in CSF yields among 90 patients:
  - 54% (+) on first lumbar puncture.
  - 82% (+) on second lumbar puncture.
  - 2–4% false (+).
  - 10–15% false (−).

- MRI is more sensitive than CT, but only picks up ∼ 2/3rds of cases, so cytology remains gold standard.
  - Patients diagnosed with leptomeningeal disease should undergo MRI of the entire neuraxis.

- Treatment:
  - 60–80% of patients will show response after intrathecal methotrexate with or without XRT.
    - Response may be durable.
    - Median survival in patients who respond is 15 months.
    - Median survival in patients who do not respond is 3–6 months.

  - XRT should be administered to symptomatic areas of leptomeningeal disease and to areas of bulky disease.
  - When you give whole brain XRT the superior retina is always included, so beware, retinopathy can develop.
  - Whole brain XRT ↑ neurotoxicity from intrathecal chemotherapy.
    - To be used only if there is cerebral or cranial nerve symptoms or if CSF flow is obstructed.
  [Mattsson W, Cancer 49: 217–220, 1982].
  - Patients receiving XRT (+) intrathecal methotrexate (via Ommaya) did better.

  [Boogerd W, Cancer 67: 1685–1695, 1991].
  - Retrospective study.

- If CSF cleared and patients improved neurologically → did better.
- If patients received concurrent systemic chemotherapy → did better.
- 11 out of 17 patients that survived longer developed leukoencephalopathy.
- Poor prognostic factors in this study:
  - Cranial nerve involvement.
  - CSF Glucose 43 or less.
  - Age > 55 years.
  - CSF Protein 51–99 mg/dl.
  - Lung metastases.

[Grossman SA, J Clin Oncol 11: 561–569, 1993].
- No advantage to combined intrathecal chemotherapy, it just ↑ toxicity.
  - ↑ leukoencephalopathy.

- Standard therapy:
  1. Intrathecal methotrexate (12 mg via reservoir) and XRT.
     - Intrathecal methotrexate two times per week × 4 weeks, then 1 time per week × 4 weeks, then every other week.
     - The most common neurologic complication of intrathecal methotrexate is a transient aseptic meningitis.
       - Develops within hours of injection.
       - Presents with headache, stiff neck, fever and confusion.
       - Does not recur with subsequent injections.

     - Systemic complications of intrathecal methotrexate.
       - Stomatitis.
       - Myelosuppression.

  2. If fails, thiotepa 10 mg/4ml, two times per week.
     - Side effects of thiotepa.
       - Myelosuppression.
       - Myelopathy.

  3. If fails, then cytarabine (ARA-C) 30 mg.

ENDOCRINE THERAPY FOR METASTATIC BREAST CANCER
[Muss HB, Breast Cancer Res Treat 21: 15–26, 1992].

- Mean time to objective response: 2 months.

- Do not change hormonal approach until after 3 months of therapy, because hormones work slowly on slowly dividing cells.

- Mean response duration: 1–2 years.

- 50% response to second hormonal treatment, if first treatment worked.

- Classically response rates to endocrine therapies are higher in patients with:
  - Postmenopause.
  - A long disease free interval.
  - No liver involvement.
  - Predominantly soft tissue metastases.
  - Slower tumor growth.
  - Older age.
  - Good response to a previous hormone therapy.

- 50–60% of ER(+) tumors respond to primary hormonal therapy.
  - If the tumor is also PR(+) the response rate rises to 70–80%.

- ER(−), PR(+) tumors respond as well to endocrine therapy as do ER(+), PR(−) cases.

- ER(−), PR(−) tumors have < 10% chance of responding to hormonal therapy.

- Successful endocrine therapy may convert a progesterone receptor positivity to negativity.

- Tumor flare.
  - Any endocrine therapy may result in tumor flare within the initial 2–4 weeks.
  - More commonly occurs in patients with skeletal metastases.
  - Usually presents with:
    1. ↑ in tumor size.

2. Bone pain.
3. Erythema of cutaneous lesions.
4. ↑ in LFT's.
5. ↑ in CEA.
6. Transitory hypercalcemia.
7. ↑ diffuse uptake on bone scan.
   - Therapy should be continued with attention given to symptom control (bone pain, hypercalcemia, etc.)
   - Symptoms resolve spontaneously within 2–3 weeks.
   - Tumor flare predicts an excellent response.

● Oophorectomy is used only in premenopausal women.

● Aminoglutethimide is only used in postmenopausal women.

● [Ingle JN, J Clin Oncol 4: 958–964, 1986].
  [Rutqvist LE, Breast Cancer Res Treat 7: 45–46, 1986].
   - Combination endocrine therapy does not offer benefit over endocrine monotherapy, just ↑ side effects.

● [Lippman ME, Cancer 46: 2829–2834, 1980].
   - Prior chemotherapy does not affect response rate to subsequent hormonal therapy.

● Generally the first choice is tamoxifen, then anastrozole, then megestrol, then aminoglutethimide.

Antiestrogens

● Tamoxifen (Nolvadex).
  [Sunderland MC, J Clin Oncol 9: 1283–1297, 1991].
   - Works in adjuvant and metastatic setting.
   - May be useful in chemoprevention.
     - For further details, refer to Chemoprevention section, page 180.
   - Tamoxifen binds to ER receptor.
     - Tamoxifen may mask the ER receptor.
   - Tamoxifen has other functions not well understood.
   - It induces apoptosis.
   - May have antiangiogenesis properties.
   - May have a cytostatic role.

- ↓ secretion of stimulatory factors (TGF-α, IGF-I, IGF-II, and PDGF).
- ↑ secretion of inhibitory growth factors (TGF-β).
- Inhibits multi-drug resistance (MDR) gene in very high doses.
- May precipitate or worsen vasomotor symptoms.
- Serum levels do not correlate with antitumor response.

- Endocrine effects:
  - Depend on age, duration, dose, and menopausal status.
  - In postmenopausal ♀—normally follicle stimulating hormone (FSH) and luteinizing hormone (LH) are increased, with tamoxifen they decrease although levels remain in normal range, these decreased levels persist at 6 and 12 months of therapy.
  - In postmenopausal ♀—on estrogen replacement the gonadotropins (FSH, LH) also decrease.
  - There is general agreement that serum estradiol and progesterone levels are unaffected by tamoxifen in postmenopausal ♀.
  - May cause paradoxical ↑ estrogen in premenopausal ♀, which may be responsible for tumor flare.
  - Approximately 50% of the patients on long term tamoxifen therapy continue to have regular ovulation and menstrual cycles; most of the rest regain menses after tamoxifen therapy is discontinued.
  - 25% patients → amenorrhea.
  - 25% patients → oligomenorrhea and irregular menses.
  - Extended duration of therapy was also associated with abnormal menses.
  - Tamoxifen induced amenorrhea was not associated with improved response rates.

  - In pre and post-menopausal ♀:
  - Antithrombin III, total cholesterol, and LDL cholesterol decrease with longterm therapy.
    - HDL cholesterol remains the same.
  - Steroid binding globulin (SHBG) is increased by tamoxifen, this protein is the major transporter for estrogenic steroids, ↑ levels of SHBG may bind and decrease plasma of free estradiol and subsequently less estrogen may be available.
  - Response to tamoxifen in premenopausal ♀ is comparable to the old literature for castration ∼ 30% response, however recent studies have improved results with castration if use ER(+) PR(+) patients.

— In the trials tamoxifen dose varies from $20 \rightarrow 120$ mg/day.
— But there is no dose response.
— Disease regression after stopping tamoxifen has been reported in the literature; all patients responded to tamoxifen initially then progressed through it.
   — All reported patients were postmenopausal.
— Patients responding to tamoxifen may show a worsening bone scan during the first 2 months due to bone healing.
— Half-life 7 days.
— Reaches steady state in 4 weeks.
— Effect on mineral density:
   [Powles TJ, J Clin Oncol 14: 78–84, 1996].
   — Randomized controlled tamoxifen chemoprevention trial done at the Royal Marsden Hospital among healthy ♀.
   — 2500 healthy ♀ randomized to placebo vs. tamoxifen 20 mg p.o. q day × 8 years.
   — Bone mineral density was reduced in premenopausal women for the first 2 years, which achieved a plateau in year number 3, but in postmenopausal women there was prevention of bone loss.
— Potential interaction between tamoxifen and coumadin.
— Serious potential interaction between tamoxifen and mitomycin.
   [Powles TJ, J Clin Oncol 13: 547–552, 1995].

— <u>SIDE EFFECTS of Tamoxifen:</u>

   — Precipitation or worsening of vasomotor symtoms.
      — Hot flashes (Pre/postmenopausal ♀).
   — Vaginal discharge/atrophic vaginitis.
   — Irregular menses.
   — Weight gain.
   — Depression, 1–2% ♀.
   — ↑ deep venous thrombosis and pulmonary embolus (DVT/PE) (very small number of patients).
      — Development of DVT does not necessarily require stopping tamoxifen.

   — Carcinogen [Smith LL, Oncology 12(3 suppl 5): 14–22, 1998].
      — Associated with endometrial cancer.

[Rutqvist LE, J Natl Cancer Inst 87: 645–651, 1995].
— In the Stockholm Breast Cancer Study Group, a higher dose (40 mg/day) was given for 2–5 years.
  — 2729 ♀ with breast cancer under the age of 71, were randomized to receive tamoxifen 40 mg/day vs. placebo.
  — Median follow-up 9 years.
  — Tamoxifen group had a 6-fold ↑ in endometrial cancer.
  — The tamoxifen group also had a 3-fold ↑ in gastro-intestinal cancers.
  — This is the only study to date that has shown an increase in gastrointestinal tract tumors in a tamoxifen treated population.

[Fisher B, J Natl Cancer Inst 86: 527–537, 1994].
— In American studies (tamoxifen 20 mg/day) there were ~ 2 cases per 1000 per year.
— NSABP-B14.
  — 2843 ♀ with LN(−)/ER(+) breast cancer.
  — Randomized to tamoxifen 20 mg/day vs. placebo.
  — Median follow-up 7 years.
  — 23 endometrial tumors found in the tamoxifen group and 2 tumors in the placebo group.

[Barakat RR, Gynecologic Oncology 55: 164–168, 1994].
— 80% of endometrial cancers associated with tamoxifen were found to be good grade disease, not bad as previously thought.
— Cerebellar (Ataxia) at very high doses.
— ↑ LFT's, reversible.
— In rats at high doses → liver cancer.
  — No cases reported in humans.
  — Dose-dependent.
  — Rat doses were equivalent to a human dose 40 mg of tamoxifen a day × 40 years.
— Hypercalcemia.
— Mild nausea.
— Mild thrombocytopenia/leukopenia.
— Ocular toxicity:
  — Retinopathy.
  — Macular edema.

- Toremifene (Fareston)
  - First antiestrogen introduced into the USA since tamoxifen.
  - 1997—FDA approval for the first-line treatment of postmenopausal women with ER(+) or ER(unknown) breast cancer.

  [Gershanovich M, Breast Cancer Res Treat, in press 1998].
  [Pyrhonen S, Br J Cancer 76(2): 270–277, 1997].
  [Gams R, Oncology 11 (6; suppl 4): 23–28, 1997].
  - Phase III trials have demonstrated that toremifene 60 mg p.o. q.d. as first-line therapy is as effective and as well tolerated as tamoxifen 20 or 40 mg/day.
  - Response duration ranges from 1.3 to > 2 years.

  [Gershanovich M, Oncology 11 (6 suppl 4): 29–36, 1997].
  - Phase III data evaluating 369 ♀ did not show any significant benefit of high doses of toremifene when compared to standard doses of tamoxifen or toremifene.

  [Saarto T, Br J Cancer 75(4): 602–605, 1997].
  - Toremifene ↓ cholesterol to a similar extent as tamoxifen, but it may also ↑ HDL cholesterol.
  - Toremifene is not genotoxic and probably has less of a proliferative effect on the endometrium than does tamoxifen.
  - SIDE EFFECTS of Toremifene:
    - Hot flashes.
    - Sweating.
    - Nausea/vomiting.
    - Vaginal discharge.
    - Dizziness.
    - Edema.
    - Vaginal bleeding.
    - LFT abnormalities.
    - Ocular changes.
    - Thromboembolic phenomena.
    - Hypercalcemia.

- Raloxifene (Evista)
  - Not indicated in the treatment of breast cancer.
  - Nonsteroidal antiestrogen.
  - Its antiproliferative activity has been demonstrated in vitro and in vivo in experimental models of breast cancer.
  - There is evidence of cross-resistance between tamoxifen and raloxifene.

– The indication for raloxifene will lie in osteoporosis therapy and potentially in chemoprevention.

Selective aromatase inhibitors
[Harvey HA, Oncology 12 (3 suppl 5): 32–35, 1998].

– Both anastrozole (1 mg/day) and letrozole (2.5 mg/day) have now been FDA approved as second-line treatment for hormone-dependent breast cancer in postmenopausal ♀ in whom the disease had progressed through tamoxifen.

– These agents have not been sufficiently tested in premenopausal ♀.
– These studies are ongoing.

● The role of intra-tumoral aromatase may be important in the treatment of breast cancer.

●· Anastrozole (Arimidex).
[Goss PE, Oncology 11: 1697–1708, 1997].
[Jonat W, Eur J Cancer 32A: 404–412, 1996].
– New selective competitive aromatase inhibitor.
– No hydrocortisone needed.
– Effective inhibitor of postmenopausal estrogen.
– Very low toxicity profile.
– Its use in premenopausal ♀ may cause a surge in gonadotropins and subsequent ↑ in estradiol levels which may be detrimental to breast cancer patients.
– In premenopausal ♀ anastrozole may be combined with LHRH agonists causing a medical castration and a complete estrogen ablation.
– Studies further evaluating this approach are ongoing.

– SIDE EFFECTS of Anastrozole:
  – GI: nausea, diarrhea.
  – Weight gain.
  – Edema.
  – Dyspnea.
  – Headache.
  – Thromboembolic disorders.
  – Hot flashes.
  – Pain.

[Buzdar A, Cancer 83: 1142–1152, 1998].

- Two Randomized clinical trials have evaluated 764 ♀ with advanced breast cancer that were progressing through antiestrogen therapy.
- These prospective Randomized multicenter trials evaluated the efficacy of:
  Anastrozole 1 mg p.o. q.d. vs.
  Anastrozole 10 mg p.o. q.d. vs.
  Megestrol acetate 40 mg p.o. qid.

- Median follow-up: 31 months.
- RESULTS:
  - ♀ receiving anastrozole experienced significantly less weight gain. Overall fewer thromboemblic events, hypertension, dyspnea, sweating and vaginal hemorrhage compared to patients receiving megestrol.
  - The study shows an improved tie to tumor progression and statistical survival advantage in ♀ treated with anastrozole 1 mg p.o. q.d.
    - Anastrozole 1 mg led to prolongation in survival of 4.2 months over megastrol acetate.

- Letrozole (Femara).
  - Third generation, non-steroidal, aromatase inhibitor.
  - 2.5 mg p.o. q.d.
  - 10 000 times as potent as aminoglutethimide in vivo.
  - No hydrocortisone needed.
  - Approved in the USA for the treatment of advanced breast cancer in postmenopausal ♀ with disease progression following antiestrogen therapy.
  - No dosage adjustment is required for renal impairment, as long as the creatinine clearance is > 10 ml/min.
  - No dosage adjustment is required for mild to moderate hepatic impairment.
    - Patients with severe hepatic impairment have not been studied.

- SIDE EFFECTS of Letrozole:
  - Musculoskeletal pain.
  - Arthralgia.
  - Nausea/vomiting.
  - Headache.

- Fatigue.
- Dyspnea.
- Weight gain.
- Vaginal bleeding.
[Smith I, 20th Annual San Antonio Breast Cancer Symposium. 1997].
- Two clinical trials were conducted, comparing two different dosages of Letrozole vs. Megestrol in one trial and vs. aminoglutethimide in the other trial.

- 1100 postmenopausal ♀ with ER(+) breast cancer or with hormonal receptor status unknown, who had not responded to tamoxifen or progressed through tamoxifen, were entered into these trials.

- In the Megestrol trial, women were Randomized to:
  Letrozole 2.5 mg p.o. q.d.
  vs.
  Letrozole 0.5 mg p.o. q.d.
  vs.
  Megestrol 160 mg p.o. q.d.

- In the Aminoglutethimide trial ♀ were Randomized to:
  Letrozole 2.5 mg p.o. q.d.
  vs.
  Letrozole 0.5 mg p.o. q.d.
  vs.
  Aminoglutethimide 250 mg p.o. b.i.d.

- Both trials have > 2 year follow-up.

- Megestrol trial:
  [Dombernowski P, J Clin Oncol 16: 453-461, 1998].
  - Double-blind Randomized trial at 91 centers in 10 countries.
  - 551 postmenopausal ♀ enrolled.
  - Response rate:
    - Letrozole 2.5 mg (24.1%).
    - Letrozole 0.5 mg (12.2%).
    - Megestrol (16.4%).
  - Median duration of response.
    - Letrozole 2.5 mg (33 months).
    - Letrozole 0.5 mg (18 months).
    - Megestrol (18 months).

— Median survival (not statistically significant).
  — Letrozole 2.5 mg (25 months).
  — Letrozole 0.5 mg (21.5 months).
  — Megestrol (21.5 months).

— Incidence of weight gain and thromboembolic phenomena were reduced in the Letrozole arms compared to the Megestrol arm.

— Aminoglutethimide trial:
  [Marty M, Proc Am Soc Clin Oncol 16: (A156) 1997].
— Randomized, not double-blind trial conducted over 2 years at 86 centers in 11 countries.
— 555 postmenopausal women were enrolled.
— Response rate: (did not differ significantly).
  — Letrozole 2.5 mg (19.5%).
  — Letrozole 0.5 mg (16.7%).
  — Aminoglutethimide (12.4%).
— Median duration of response.
  — Letrozole 2.5 mg (21 months).
  — Letrozole 0.5 mg (18 months).
  — Aminoglutethimide (14 months).
— Overall survival.
  — Favored the 2.5 mg Letrozole arm.
  — Both doses of Letrozole proved to be more active against visceral lesions with objective response rates of 19 and 17% compared to 3% for aminoglutethimide.
  — Incidence of rash was 3% in the Letrozole arms vs. 12% in the aminoglutethimide arms.

● Vorozole (Rizivor).
  [Johnston SR, Cancer Res 54: 5875–5881, 1994].
  — New selective aromatase inhibitor.
  — No hydrocortisone needed.
  — Only to be used in postmenopausal women.
  [Goss PE, Proc Am Soc Clin Oncol 16: (A542) 1997].
  — Preliminary reports from studies comparing vorozole to megestrol and aminoglutethimide show a therapeutic advantage for vorozole.
  — Not yet approved for clinical use.
  — SIDE EFFECTS of Vorozole:
    — Hot flashes.
    — Headaches.
    — Nausea.

● 4-hydroxyandrostenedione (Formestane).
  [Coombes RC, Eur J Cancer 28a:1941–1945, 1992].
  – Highly selective aromatase inhibitor.
  – Commercially available in Europe.
  – Its use is somewhat limited by its associated injection site reactions.
  – Produces an objective response rate of 24–35% in the first-line treatment of advanced breast cancer.

Non-selective aromatase inhibitors

● Aminoglutethimide (Cytadren).
  – Non-selective aromatase (estrogen synthetase) inhibitor.
  – Causes a medical adrenalectomy by blocking the conversion of adrenal androgens to estrogens.
  – 1 gm q.d. with 40 mg hydrocortisone.
  – At standard doses, administer with hydrocortisone to avoid hypocortisolism.
  – Response rate same as tamoxifen.
  – Administer only to postmenopausal ♀.
  – [Cocconi G, J Clin Oncol 10: 984–989, 1992].
    – 250 mg p.o. b.i.d. without hydrocortisone is as effective as 1000 mg (250 mg qid) p.o. with 20 mg p.o. b.i.d. hydrocortisone, which has been the standard for years.
  – CONCLUSION:
    – Low dose as good as standard dose.
  – SIDE EFFECTS of Aminoglutethimide:
    – Lethargy/Ataxia (often disappears in ∼ 4 weeks).
    – Mental status changes: sedation, dizziness.
    – Fever.
    – Macular rash.
      – Usually resolves in 1–2 weeks.
      – May progress to Stevens–Johnson syndrome.
    – Hypothyroidism.
    – Leukopenia (Agranulocytosis).
    – Anorexia.
    – Dizziness.
    – Thrombocytopenia (prolonged).
    – Lupus-like syndrome.

Progestational agents

- Megestrol Acetate (Megace).
  - 40 mg p.o. qid or 80 mg p.o. bid.
  - SIDE EFFECTS of Megace:
    - Weight gain.
    - ↑ pulmonary embolus and deep venous thrombosis.

GnRH analogs (gonadotropin hormone-releasing analogs)
[Blamey RW, Eur J Cancer 28a: 810–14, 1992].

- Goserelin acetate (Zoladex).
  - Used as in prostate cancer, administered monthly by injection.

- Leuprolide acetate (Lupron).
  - Used as in prostate cancer, administered monthly by injection.

- These compounds bind to luteinizing hormone-releasing hormone (LHRH) receptors in the pituitary causing a ↓ in estrogen to castration levels.
- Breast tumors contain LHRH receptors.
- Tumor responses reported in ER(+) and ER(−) patients.
  - Responses are higher with ER(+) tumors.
  [Kaufmann M, J Clin Oncol 7: 1113–1119, 1989].
- Work best in premenopausal ♀ with advanced disease.
- Switch off the hypothalamic–pituitary axis which in turn switches off the ovaries.
- Approved for premenopausal patients, responses also reported in some postmenopausal patients. [Saphner T, J Clin Oncol 11: 1529–1535, 1993]
- Prevent compensatory ↑ in estradiol in premenopausal women.
- Cause a medical oophorectomy.
  - Objective response rates in the range of 40% have been reported in ♀ with advanced disease.
  [Kimmick G, Oncology 9: 877–890, 1995].
  - There are case reports of premenopausal ♀ responding to oophorectomy after progressing through LHRH agonists.
  [Williams MR, Br J Cancer 53: 629–636, 1986].

- Avoid the psychological trauma and operative morbidity of the of the irreversible operative castration.

– SIDE EFFECTS of GnRH analogs:
  – Injection site reaction.
  – Tumor flare.
  – Hot flashes.
  – Loss of libido in premenopausal patients.

Oophorectomy

● Ovarian ablation.
  – Has been around for ~ 100 years.
  – It works!
  – The question that remains is when to use it and how.

● For its effect in ♀ younger than 50 years of age, with early breast cancer, please refer to the Oxford Overview Study by the Early Breast Cancer Trialists Collaborative Group. on page 90.

● [Pritchard KI, Cancer Treat Rep 64: 787–796, 1980].
  [Sawka CA Cancer Res 46: 3152–3156, 1986].
  – The response to tamoxifen predicted response to castration.

● [Hoogstraten B, Cancer Res 42: 4788–4791, 1982].
  – The SWOG study did not support this finding. Instead it concluded that patients who were tamoxifen failures responded to oophorectomy.

● Phase III clinical trials in premenopausal ♀.
  – Two Randomized prospective trials compared tamoxifen vs. oophorectomy (surgical)
  a. British study [Buchanan RB, J Clin Oncol 4: 1326–1330, 1986]
     – 122 ♀ randomized to tamoxifen vs. surgical castration as initial therapy for metastatic disease.
     – ER status not checked in these patients (major flaw of study).
     – Tamoxifen patients → 24% response rate for 20 months duration.
     – Castration patients → 21% response rate for 7 months duration.
     – Not statistically significant: median survival greater in oophorectomy group, but not significantly.
  b. Mayo Clinic Study [Ingle JN, J Clin Oncol 4: 178–185, 1986].
     – 54 only ER(+) ♀ entered but only 80% of ER status was known.

- Oophorectomy → 35% response rate.
- Tamoxifen → 27% response rate.
- No significant difference in duration of response or survival.

● Surgical or medical oophorectomy is clearly efficacious as adjuvant hormonal therapy in premenopausal ♀.

● Laparoscopic oophorectomy is an emerging option, once oophorectomy has been chosen. [Walsh D, The Breast 7: 150–153, 1998].

● The Scottish Trial.
   [SCTBG, Lancet 341: 1293–1298, 1993].
   - Premenopausal ♀ with early breast cancer.
   - CMF vs. ovarian ablation.
   - Overall relapse-free and overall survival for the two groups were identical.
      - Point of interest:
         - ♀ with ER(+) tumors had a better DFS and OS with oophorectomy.
         - ♀ with ER(−) tumors had a better DFS and OS with CMF chemotherapy.

● The Intergroup has just completed a study evaluating the effect of ovarian ablation after the administration of chemotherapy.
   - The three arms after chemotherapy were:
      a. Zoladex.
      b. Zoladex/Tamoxifen.
      c. Observation.

STANDARD CHEMOTHERAPY FOR METASTATIC BREAST CANCER

[J Clin Oncol 14(8): 2197–2205, 1996].

- In a large series of patients treated with the standard chemotherapy regimens at MD Anderson Hospital, ∼ 17% of the patients achieved a CR and only 3% remained in remission > 5 years.

- Standard chemotherapy for metastatic breast cancer will result in ∼ 10–20% complete response (CR) in HR(−) ♀.

- Time to disease progression with standard chemotherapy ranges from 4–9 months with median survival of 12–16 months.

- Duration of chemotherapy in the metastatic setting.
  [Muss HB, New Engl J Med 325: 1342–1348, 1991].
  [Coates A, New Engl J Med 317: 1490–1495, 1987].
  − Therapy is continued as long as disease is present.
  − Continuous therapy seems to improve quality of life among these ♀.

- Factors that predict response to chemotherapy.
  [Falkson G, J Clin Oncol 9: 2153–2161, 1991].
  − High proliferative index.
  − Premenopausal status.
  − Prolonged disease free interval.
  − Good performance status.
  − Presence of visceral involvement.
  − Presence of two or more metastatic sites.

- Doxorubicin (Adriamycin) and Epidoxorubicin (Epirubicin).
  − Considered to be the most active single agents, with response rates in excess of 40% in previously untreated ♀.
  − In combination regimens, response rates range up to 70%.
  − In second-line treatment of metastatic breast cancer, response rates have ranged from 25–33%, with a median time to progression of 3.6 months, and a median survival of 8.9 months. [Henderson IC, J Clin Oncol 7: 560–571, 1989].

- CAF/AC/CMF.
  - CAF or FAC.
    - Cyclophosphamide 400–600 mg/m^2 i.v. day 1.
    - Adriamycin 40–60 mg/m^2 i.v. day 1 (may be given by c.i. 48–96 h).
    - Fluorouracil 400–600 mg/m^2 i.v. day 1 (can also be given day 1, 8).
    - Repeat cycle q 21 days (or q 28 days, if used with above regimens in the parentheses).
  - AC.
    - Adriamycin 60 mg/m^2 i.v. day 1.
    - Cyclophosphamide 600 mg/m^2 i.v. day 1.
    - Repeat cycle q 21 days.
  - CMF.
    - Cyclophosphamide 100 mg/m^2 p.o. days 1 through 14 or 400–600 mg/m^2 i.v. day 1.
    - Methotrexate 40–60 mg/m^2 i.v. days 1 and 8.
    - Fluorouracil 400–600 mg/m^2 i.v. days 1 and 8.
    - Repeat cycle q 28 days.

- CMF may have a role even if previously used as adjuvant therapy, it can be successfully used again, if the disease free survival is in excess of 12 months.
  [3rd International Conference on Adjuvant Therapy of Breast Cancer; March 2–5, 1988, St. Gallen, Switzerland].
  - Valagussa reported 29 patients at the National Cancer Institute of Milan, who received CMF again at relapse but had had a disease-free interval of > 12 months. The response rate was 41% with a median response of 18 months. These patients were compared with those who had relapsed after having been previously randomized for treatment with radical mastectomy alone. Of these, 45 received CMF and 38% responded with a median response duration of 16 months.
  - Similar data have been reported with FAC after FAC.

  - SIDE EFFECTS of CMF:
  - Cyclophosphamide (Cytoxan).
    - Hemorrhagic cystitis.
      - Due to acrolein, a metabolite that accumulates in the bladder.
  - Methotrexate (Folex).
    - Excreted via kidney, follow renal function.

- Liver toxicity.
- Distributes slowly into pleural and ascitic fluid.
- Fluorouracil (Adrucil).
- Mucositis.
- Palmar/plantar erythromelalgia (hand/foot syndrome).
- Acute and chronic conjunctivitis.
- Cerebellar ataxia.

● Taxanes.
  [D'Andrea GM, Seminars in Oncology 24(4 suppl 13): 27–44, 1997].
  - Taxol and Taxotere.
  - The optimal dose, schedule, and combination chemotherapy has yet to be identified for either taxane.

● Paclitaxel (Taxol).
  [Seidman AD, J Clin Oncol 13: 1152–1159, 1995].
  [Helson L, Cancer Investigation 12(1): 30–33, 1994].
  - Antimicrotubule agent from the bark of the western Pacific yew (*Taxus brevifolia*).
  - Promotes and stabilizes microtubule assembly and inhibits depolymerization in contrast to vinca alkaloids (vincristine, vinblastine, navelbine) and colchicine, which cause microtubule disassembly.
  - Phase II studies have documented response rates in metastatic breast cancer ranging from 28 to 62%, depending on extent of prior therapy.
    - Active agent in metastatic patients with refractory disease.
  - The studies done with refractory patients show response > 50%.
  - MD Anderson reported in untreated metastatic patients, > 60% response rate.

  - Taxol response in metastatic breast cancer.
    - In adriamycin virgins → ~ 60%.
    - Not adriamycin virgins → ~ 20–30%.
    - Refractory to adriamycin → < 20%.

1. Memorial Study (MSK).
   [Nabholtz JM, Proc Am Soc Clin Oncol 12: 60 (A42)1993].
   - 72 patients (after 2 prior regimens).
   - 50% of these were anthracycline resistant; that is relapsed within 12 months of anthracycline therapy.
   - Overall partial response of 72 patients → 28%.
   - Myelosuppression dose limiting toxicity.

2. Europe study.
   — 3-h regimen.
   — Overall response → ∼ 30%.
   — Pre-medicate (dexamethasone, benadryl, cimetidine).
   — With 3-h infusion vs. 24-h infusion as dose ↑; the dose limiting toxicity is neurotoxicity not myelosuppression.
3. [Nabholtz JM, J Clin Oncol 14(6): 1858–1867, 1996].
   — 471 ♀ with metastatic breast cancer, previously treated, were Randomized.
   Group I: Taxol 175 mg/m²/3-h infusion q 3 weeks, vs.
   Group II: Taxol 135 mg/m²/3-h infusion q 3 weeks.
   — RESULTS:
     — Overall response rate:
       — Group I → 29%.
       — Group II → 22% ($P = 0.108$).
     — Complete response:
       — Group I → 5%.
       — Group II → 2% ($P = 0.088$).
     — Median time to disease progression:
       — Group I → 4.2 months.
       — Group II → 3 months.
     — Median survival time:
       — Group I → 11.7 months.
       — Group II → 10.5 months.

   — Incidence and severity of neutropenia and peripheral neuropathy were dose related.

   — The most commonly used dose of paclitaxel today is 175 mg/m² over 3 h q 3 weeks. This displays a complete and partial response rate of ∼ 30% in previously treated MBC with a median time to progression of 4–5 months after therapy started.

4. NSABP-B26
   [Mamounas E, Proc Am Soc Clin Oncol 17: A389, 1998].
   — 563 ♀ with stage IIIb (16%) and stage IV (84%) breast cancer were Randomized to two different Taxol infusion regimens.
   Group I (276 ♀) Taxol 250 mg/m² 3-h infusion
                              vs.
   Group II (278 ♀) Taxol 250 mg/m² 24-h infusion.

- Preliminary RESULTS:
  - 11 possibly or probably related treatment deaths.
  - 7 from group I and 4 from group II.
- Group II had:
  - ↑ hematological toxicity
  - ↓ neurosensory toxicity.
- Had a higher tumor response rate
- Multivariate analysis did not detect significant differences in treatment effect at age, stage, and prior adjuvant chemotherapy.

5. CALGB 9342.
- Ongoing trial.
- Evaluating three different doses of Taxol in previously treated ♀.
- ♀ are Randomized to:
  Taxol 175 mg/m² vs. Taxol 210 mg/m² vs. Taxol 250 mg/m².
- All Taxol is given in a 3 h i.v. infusion and cycles are repeated every 21 days.

6. Intergroup Study E 1193.
  [Sledge GW, Proc Am Soc Clin Oncol 16: 2, 1997].
- ♀ with metastatic breast cancer were assigned to single agent therapy.
- There was crossover among single agent arms at the time of progression.
- ♀ Randomized to:
  Paclitaxel 175 mg/m²/24-h infusion (229 ♀) vs.
  Doxorubicin 60 mg/m² (224 ♀) vs.
  Paclitaxel at 150 mg/m²/24-h infusion and doxorubicin at 50 mg/m² (230 ♀).
- Every regimen was given q. 3 weeks.
- In the combined arm paclitaxel was given 4-h after doxorubicin and by 24-h infusion and with granulocyte colony stimulating factor support.

- Response rates:
  - 34% single agent doxorubicin.
  - 33% single agent placitaxel.
  - 46% for combined therapy.
- Median time to treatment failure was 2 months longer in the combined arm. (8 vs. 6 months).
- No significant difference in survival or in quality of life was noted between the 3 arms.

7. EORTC 10961.
   – Ongoing trial
   – Phase III Randomized trial evaluating doxorubicin/paclitaxel vs. doxorubicin/cyclophosphamide in previously untreated ♀ with metastatic breast cancer.

8. A Randomized trial comparing paclitaxel and docetaxel is currently underway.

– Taxanes and navelbine together have also been shown to be active combinations.

– When using taxol with platinum, give taxol first to ameliorate neutropenia.

– When using taxol with cyclophosphamide, give taxol first to ameliorate the neutropenia.

– When using taxol with adriamycin, give adriamycin first to ameliorate the neutropenia.
   [Holmes FA, J Clin Oncol 14: 2713–2721, 1996].
   [Gianni L, J Clin Oncol 15: 1906–1915, 1997].
   – Paclitaxel whether administered over 3 h or over 24 h ↓ doxorubicin clearance; this may explain the ↑ cardiac toxicity reported with this combination as well as the antitumor activity.

– Phenobarbitol and dilantin ↑ the metabolism of taxol, so ↓ plasma levels of taxol.

– SIDE EFFECTS of Paclitaxel:
   – Myelosuppression; neutropenia.
   – Peripheral neuropathy.
      – Rare when < 170 mg/m^2 are used.
   – Hypersensitivity reactions.
      – Premedicate with steroids, benadryl and H2 blockers.
      – 2 sudden deaths reported in Memorial Phase I study.
      – May be secondary to cremaphor, the transport vehicle for the drug.
      – Rash, urticaria, dyspnea.
      – With 24-h infusion, hypersensitivity reactions decreased in intensity.

- Cardiac toxicity.
- May be secondary to hypersensitivity reaction.
- Alopecia, myalgia/arthralgia.
- Mucositis, nausea/vomiting.
- Typhlitis [Pestalozzi BC, Cancer 71: 1797–1800, 1993].
  - Reported in two patients who received taxol 180 mg/m² and doxorubicin 75 mg/m² given simultaneously in a 72° continuous infusion (c.i.) followed by G-CSF. Both patients did well with conservative treatment and were retreated successfully with taxol 160 mg/m² and doxorubicin 60 mg/m² with G-CSF.

- Docetaxel (Taxotere).
  [Hortobagyi GN, Oncology 11(8): 11–41, 1997].
  [Trudeau ME, Semin Oncol 22(2:suppl 4): 17–21, 1995].
  [Trudeau M, Cancer Investigation 12(1): 35–36, 1994].
  [Piccart MJ ASCO Highlights: 25–32, 1993].
  - From needles of European yew tree (*Taxus baccata*).
  - Same mechanism of action as Taxol.
  - Standard dose 60–100 mg/m² i.v. over 1 h q 21 days.

  - 90% of the drug is metabolized by the liver.
    - Do not give if AST and/or ALT is > 1.5 (the upper limit of normal) and concomitantly the alkaline phosphatase is > 2.5 (the upper limit of normal).

  - Phase II studies: 100 mg/m² i.v. over 1–2 h q 21 days.
    [Gradisher WJ, Oncology 11(8): 15–18, 1997].
    [Trudeau ME, Anticancer Drugs 7(Suppl 2): 9–12, 1996].
    - 5-phase II studies in breast cancer have been done.
    - As a first line chemotherapy for stage III and metastatic breast cancer, response rates up to 68%.

  [Ravdin PM, J Clin Oncol 13: 2879–2885, 1995].
  [Eisenhauer EA, Eur J Cancer 31A Suppl 4: S11–13, 1995].
  [Valero V, J Clin Oncol 13: 2886–2894, 1994].
  - Three multicenter studies show that single-agent docetaxel in anthracycline-resistant patients produces a response rate of ∼41% and a median survival of 10 months.

  - May have more activity than Taxol in patients with anthracycline-resistant disease.
    - A direct phase III comparison study is going on.

[Chan S, Oncology (Suppl 8): 19–24, 1997].
[Chan S, Proc Am Soc Clin Oncol 16: 154, 1997].
— Nonblinded, multicenter, Randomized phase III trial.
— 326 pre and postmenopausal ♀ in whom previous alkylating therapy failed.
— No previous anthracycline, anthracenedione, or taxane therapy was permitted.
— ♀ Randomized to:
  — Docetaxel 100 mg/m^2 over 1 h q 3 weeks vs.
  — Doxorubicin 75 mg/m^2 for 15–20 min q 3 weeks.

Preliminary data of 200 women		
	Docetaxel (%)	Doxorubicin (%)
Median time to progression	29 weeks	21 weeks
Overall response rate	47	27
Complete response	10	3
Progressive disease	10	22
Grade IV neutropenia	78	81
Grade III/IV thrombocytopenia	1	16.9
Neurotoxicity	5	0

[ASCO Highlights: 1996].
— 36 patients evaluated.
— Ongoing trial.
— Dose: 100 mg/m^2 i.v. q 21 days.
— Premedicated with dexamethasone 8 mg p.o. bid, days 1–4.

— CONCLUSION: preliminary reports show taxotere has antitumor activity in patients with taxol-resistant metastatic breast cancer previously exposed to anthracyclines.

— SIDE EFFECTS of Docetaxel:
  — Myelosuppression-limiting dose toxicity.
    — Neutropenia: day 4–day 7.

— Mucositis.
  — Goes along with neutropenia.

— Capillary leak syndrome.
  — Very high incidence of severe edema → peripheral and pleural effusion (not cardiac).
  — Occurs if patients are not premedicated.
  — 12/24 responding patients in EORTC study for breast cancer developed it.

— Corresponds to 400 mg total dose which corresponds to fourth to fifth cycle.
  — By 500 mg dose, 80% of the patients had some edema.
  — Steroid premedication reduces the incidence of severe fluid retention to ≤ 10%.
  — Premedicate patients with five doses of 8 mg of dexamethasone p.o. b.i.d. × 2.5 days, beginning 24 h before the treatment.

— Hypersensitivity reactions reported.
— No cardiac toxicity to date.
— Skin toxicity.
  — Macular papular rash with desquamation.
  — If it occurs, it is usually with the first cycle, does not recur.
  — Nail changes.

— Nausea, diarrhea.
— Neurotoxicity.
  — Numbness, weakness.
  — Burning dysaesthesias.
    — Pyridoxine may help with symptoms.

— Asthenia.
— Alopecia.
  — In 80% of patients.

● Mitoxantrone (Novantrone).
  — Anthraquinone derivative of doxorubicin.
  — Less effective than adriamycin.
  — Less cardiac toxicity than adriamycin.
    — Cardiac effects seen with cumulative dosing.

— Cardiac toxicity of mitoxantrone is additive to the cardiac toxicity of doxorubicin.

[Harris AL, Lancet 335: 186–190, 1990].
[Stein M, Oncology 48: 265–269, 1991].
— Mitoxantrone (14 mg/m^2 q 3 week) vs. Adriamycin.
— Dose limiting toxicity → myelosuppression.
— Less hair loss, less nausea, vomiting and mucositis than with adriamycin.
— Less heart toxicity than with adriamycin.
— > 150 mg/m^2 worry about heart toxicity.
— Dose intense mitoxantrone > 40 mg/m^2 per cycle + GCSF is currently being studied at UCSF.
— May see bluish discoloration of sclerae, fingernails and urine.

[Hainsworth JD, J Clin Oncol 9 (10): 1731–1735, 1991].
— Mitoxantrone 12 mg/m^2 on day 1 only.
— 5FU 3500 mg/m^2 i.v. push on days 1, 2, and 3.
— After the 5FU, give 300 mg i.v. leucovorin over 1 h on days 1, 2, and 3.
— 65% overall response rate in 31 women, of whom 58% had already received one metastatic regimen.
— Toxicity: myelosuppression.

- Epirubicin.
  [Robert J, Drugs 45: 20–30, 1993].
  [Periti P, Cancer Invest 9: 249–255, 1991].
  — Semisynthetic doxorubicin stereoisomer.
  — Used extensively in Europe.
  — Pending FDA approval in U.S. for 1999.
  — Single agent response rate is comparable to doxorubicin.
  — Frequently used in combination regimens with 5FU and cyclophosphamide.
    — FEC regimen.
  — Standard dose is 75–90 mg/m^2 i.v. q 3 weeks when used alone.
  — Standard dose is 60 mg/m^2 i.v. q 3 weeks when used in combination therapy.

  — SIDE EFFECTS of Epirubicin:
    — Dose limiting toxicity—myelosuppression.

- Cumulative dose-related toxicity → cardiac. See page 138.
  - Reported to have less cardiac toxicity than doxorubicin.
- Mucositis.
- Nausea and vomiting.
- Reversible alopecia.

● 5FU.
  [Chang AY, Am J Clin Oncol 12: 453–455, 1989].
  - Continuous infusion (175–250 mg/m^2/day) everyday.
  - 30–35% response in refractory women.
  - Not myelo-suppressive.
  - SIDE EFFECTS of 5FU:
    - Mucositis, hand/foot syndrome.
    - Diarrhea.
    - Cerebellar ataxia.

● 5FU/Leucovorin.
  [Loprinzi CL, Am J Clin Oncol 14: 30–32, 1991].
  - Responses have been reported in patients whose previous therapy with 5FU had failed.

● Methotrexate/Leucovorin.
  [Jolivet J, New Engl J Med 309: 1094–1104, 1983].
  - 250 mg/m^2 i.v. days 1 through 3.

● Vinorelbine (Navelbine).
  [Vogel CL, Cancer Investigation 12(1): 17–18, 1994].
  [Smith GA, Oncology 9(8): 767–773, 1995].
  - Not FDA approved for the treatment of breast cancer.

  - Semi-synthetic vinka alkaloid.
    - Inhibits microtubule polymerization.
    - Arrests the cells in metaphase.
  - Five studies from Europe and South America and one from the USA have used single agent navelbine in 310 patients with no prior chemotherapy for metastatic breast cancer.
    - Response rate 43–52%.

  - Intravenous navelbine weekly as 2nd and 3rd line agent was tried in 117 patients.
    - Response rate 17–30%.

- 30 mg/m^2 i.v. q week, until progression.

- Good for chest wall recurrence.

- Metabolized mainly by the liver.
  - Dose reduction is recommended if liver function abnormalities are present.

[Weber BL, J Clin Oncol 13: 2722–2730, 1995].
- 107 ♀ with advanced breast cancer were evaluated.
- Multicenter nonrandomized open-label phase II study.
- Patients who have previously received an anthracycline or a vinca alkaloid in the previous 12 months were excluded from the study.
- 30 mg/m^2 i.v. q week was given until progression.
- The objective response:
  - 35% for first line patients.
  - 32% for second line patients.
- Median duration of objective response was 34 weeks in both groups.
- Overall survival duration:
  - 67 weeks for first line patients.
  - 62 weeks for second line patients.
- Granulocytopenia was the dose-limiting toxicity.
- This study confirmed the finding of previous international studies.

- SIDE EFFECTS of Vinorelbine:
  - Myelosuppression.
    - Granulocytopenia-dose limiting toxicity.
      - Nadir occurs at 7–10 days, with recovery 1–2 weeks later.
    - Thrombocytopenia.
      - Rare to see platelet counts < 100000 (seen in ∼ 10% of the patients).
    - Anemia, mild.
  - GI: Nausea, vomiting, constipation and diarrhea.
  - Vesicant (mild).
  - Alopecia occurs rarely, ∼ 12% of patients.
  - Neurotoxicity—rare.
    - Low affinity for axonal microtubules may explain low incidence of neurotoxicity.
    - Incidence of neurotoxicity is lower than with vincristine or vinblastine.

— Reversible paresthesias or hypoaesthesias in ~ 30% of ♀.
— Dyspnea occurs in ~ 9% of ♀ within hours after the administration.
— Probably an allergic reaction.

- 5FU/Navelbine.
  [Dieras V, J Clin Oncol 14(12): 3097–3104, 1996].
  — 63 ♀ with advanced breast cancer were entered into this phase II trial.
  — Regimen:
    — 5FU 750 mg/m²/day c.i. × 5 days, and
    — Navelbine 30 mg/m² on day 1 and day 5 as a short i.v. infusion, every three weeks.
  — Treatment was given on an outpatient basis in the majority of the cases.
  — RESULTS:
    — 41/63 ♀ achieved an objective response.
      — Response rate was 61.6%.
    — Response rate did not differ significantly according to:
      — Type of prior adjuvant therapy.
      — Site of metastatic disease.
      — Number of metastatic sites.
    — Median response duration was 12.3 months.
    — Median overall survival was 23 months, and 28 months for the patients who had achieved a CR.

  — SIDE EFFECTS of 5FU/Navelbine:
    — Neutropenia (90% of the patients).
    — Infection (12.7% of the patients).
    — Mucositis (37% of the patients).
    — Constipation (95% of the patients).

- Velban (Vinblastine).
  [Fraschini G, Cancer 56: 225–229, 1985].
  — Vinca alkaloid.
  — Continuous infusion × 5 days.
  — 1.5 mg/m²/day.
    — Toxicity: myelosuppression.

- Mitomycin/Velban.
  — Second or third line treatment for metastatic disease.
  — Mitomycin 20 mg/m² day 1.
    — Beware of secondary hemolytic-uremic-syndrome.

- Velban 1.5 mg/m^2 days 1 and 21.
- Repeat cycle q 6–8 weeks.
- Serious interaction between mitomycin and tamoxifen.

- VATH: Velban, Adriamycin, Thiotepa, Halotestin (fluoxymesterone).
  [Hart RD, Cancer 48: 1522–1527, 1981].
  - Vinblastine 4.5 mg/m^2 i.v. day 1.
  - Doxorubicin 45 mg/m^2 i.v. day 1.
  - Thiotepa 12 mg/m^2 i.v. day 1.
  - Repeat q 21 days.
  - Fluoxymesterone 30 mg. p.o.q. day through all courses.

- Cisplatin (Platinol).
  - 30 mg/m^2, q.d. × 4 days q 3 weeks.

- Cisplatin/Etoposide.
  [Cocconi G, J Clin Oncol 9: 664–669, 1991].
  - Cisplatin 20–33 mg/m^2 days 1 through 5.
  - Etoposide 60–100 mg/m^2 days 1 through 5.

- Carboplatin (Paraplatin).
  [Crown J, Cancer 71: 1254–1257, 1993].
  - Carboplatin has a lower response rate than cisplatin.

SIDE EFFECTS of CHEMOTHERAPY:

- Generally well tolerated.

- Alopecia:
  - Seen in all cases of adriamycin, taxol, and taxotere.
  - Seen in about ~ 50% of cases of cyclophosphamide.

- Cardiac toxicity:
  - Doxorubicin (Adriamycin).
  - Congestive heart failure.
    - < 1% ♀ whose total dose is < 320 mg/m^2.
    - 1–10% ♀ whose total dose is 550 mg/m^2.
  - Cardiac arrhythmias.
  - Hours to days after administration.
  - [Hortobagyi GN, Cancer 63: 37–45, 1989].
    - 48–96-h continuous infusion schedules of adriamycin significantly ↓ the risk of cardiac toxicity.
    [Speyer JL, J Clin Oncol 10: 117–127, 1992].
  - ADR-529 (ICRF-187).
  - Provides significant cardio protection.
  - Primary toxicity is neutropenia.

  - Epirubicin.
  - Congestive heart failure.
    - 5–10% ♀ whose total dose is 1000 mg/m^2.

  - Mitoxantrone (Novantrone).
  [Unverferth DV, Cancer Treat Rep 67: 343–350, 1983].
  - Cardiac side effects are seen with cumulative dosing.
  - The 1–10% incidence of cardiac toxicity, which occurs with doxorubicin at ~ 550 mg/m^2 is found with mitoxantrone at ~ 150 mg/m^2.
  - Its cardiac toxicity is additive to that of doxorubicin.

  - 5FU.
  [de Forni M, J Clin Oncol 10: 1795–1801, 1992].
  - Cardiac toxicity appears to be ↑ in patients treated with continuous infusion 5FU.
  - Prospective study.

- 367 ♀ patients with chemotherapy regimens that included 600–1000 mg/m² per day, by 96 or 120 h continuous infusion.
- Angina pectoris, hypotension, hypertension, arrhythmias, and sudden death occurred in 7.6% of patients.

- Weight gain (> 20%):
  - Occurs in up to 40% of the ♀.

- Extravasation:
  - Be careful, especially with vesicants like doxorubicin, mitomycin-C, vinblastine, vincristine, and vinorelbine.
  - Lesions are slow to heal and difficult to graft.

- Thrombotic events:
  - Both venous and arterial, are increased by adjuvant chemotherapy, even when prednisone and tamoxifen are 'not' part of the regimen.

- Fatigue.

- Febrile/neutropenia:
  - Rare.

- Amenorrhea/infertility:
  - Age related.
  - Current CMF schedules disrupt the menstrual cycle temporarily.
  - Approximately one-third of patients become postmenopausal.
    - Most ♀ < 30 years of age continue to menstruate during and after chemotherapy.
    - ∼ 90% of ♀ > 40 years of age become permanently amenorrheic.

- Hot flashes:
  - For more details refer to section, Menopausal symptoms on page 156.
  - Whether they are secondary to chemotherapy or tamoxifen, the following measures may be effective:
  - Vitamin E 800 units every day.
    - Try for a month before calling it a failure.
  - Clonidine patches of 0.1–0.2 mg q.d. (works approximately in 40% of patients.

  - Anticholinergics—belladonna.

- Acute Leukemia (AL)/ Myelodysplastic syndrome (MDS):
  [Damandidou E, J Clin Oncol 14: 2722–2730, 1996].
  [Curtis RE, New Engl J Med 326(26): 1745–1751, 1992].
  – Factors that ↑ the risk of developing AL/MDS.
  – Use of multiple alkylating agents.
  – Duration of therapy.
  – Use of combination radiation therapy and chemotherapy.
  – Age < 50.
  – Cumulative dose of alkylating agents.

  [Fisher B, J Clin Oncol 3: 1640–1658, 1985].
  – The NSABP experience.
  – Woman at highest risk were treated with multiple alkylating agents
    and regional radiotherapy.
  – 1.3% incidence at 7 years.

  [DeCillis A. 20th Annual San Antonio Breast Cancer Symposium. 1997].
  [DeCillis A. Proc Am Soc Clin Oncol 16: 459, 1997].
  – NSABP-B25.
    – Among 2548 ♀ enrolled in NSABP-B25, there were 12 cases of AL
      and 4 cases of myelodysplasia.
    – The estimated 4-year incidence of AL/MDS was 0.87% for the
      entire study population, higher than expected on the basis of
      previous NSABP trials.

  – Dose intense CEF study.
    – Please refer to page 94.
    – To date five cases of acute leukemia have been reported in the
      dose-intense CEF arm while none have been reported in the
      standard CMF arm.

  – Radiation.
    – Risks are increased slightly by post mastectomy chest wall radia-
      tion involving the bone marrow.

  – Alkylators.
    – Drug induced leukemia appears to be an early effect, soon after
      exposure; the excess risk decreases ~ 7–10 years after exposure.
      – No cases of chronic myelogenous leukemia (CML) or acute
        lymphocytic leukemia (ALL) reported.

- Women treated with alkylating agents had an 8-fold increase in risk of acute myelogenous leukemia/ myelodysplastic syndrome (AL/MDS).
  - Erythroleukemia is a classic leukemia to follow alkylators.
  - L-phenylalanine mustard (melphalan) is 10 × more leukogenic than cyclophosphamide.
  - After 350 mg cumulative dose of melphalan, an increased risk of 100-fold.
  - Risk with cyclophosphamide increases markedly after 20000 mg.
  - 5/10000 ♀ at 10 years with cyclophosphamide doses used today.

- Cognitive impairment:

  [Yaffe K, J Am Med Assoc 279: 688–695, 1998].
  - There is some evidence that estrogen therapy improves cognitive performance in recently menopausal ♀, but no evidence of a beneficial effect in asymptomatic ♀.
  - The use of estrogen replacement therapy among breast cancer survivors remains a heated topic of controversy and should only be used in a Randomized clinical trial.

  [van Dam FSAM, J Natl Cancer Inst 90: 210–218, 1998].
  - The Netherland Group evaluated the adverse effects of chemotherapy on cognitive function.
  - Three groups of ♀, all younger than 55 years and with breast cancer were evaluated.

    - Group I: control group (34 ♀).
      - Stage I breast cancer.
      - Received no adjuvant therapy.

    - Group II: 34 ♀.
      - Stage II/III breast cancer ≥ 4 (+)LN.
      - Received four cycles of FEC (5FU, epirubicin, cyclophosphamide) followed by locoregional XRT and tamoxifen 40 mg p.o. qd × 3 years.

    - Group III: 36 ♀.
      - Stage II/III breast cancer ≥ 4 (+)LN.

- Received four cycles of FEC chemotherapy (as above) followed by a cycle of high-dose therapy with autologous stem cell rescue, locoregional XRT and tamoxifen 40 mg p.o. qd × 2 years.
- ♀ were assessed a minimum of 6 months after completion of hormonal therapy with a battery of neuropsychologic testing.
- Cognitive impairment was detected in:
  - Group I → 9%.
  - Group II → 17%.
  - Group III → 32%.
- It is not clear whether the level of cognitive impairment they experienced actually interfered with normal functioning.
- Depression and fatigue were more common in the high-dose arm (Group III).
- The study suggests a dose-response effect where more intense therapy elicits greater deficits.

Investigational agents
- High-dose therapy.
  - Randomized trials are ongoing.
  - For details, please refer to the next section: high-dose therapy.

- Anti-angiogenesis therapy.
  [Twardowski P, Current Opinion in Oncology 9(6): 584–589, 1997].
  [Folkman J, New Engl J Med 333: 1757–1763, 1995].
  - Angiogenesis is a necessary step in the growth of cancer and the development of its metastases.
  - Endothelial cells secrete many proteins that act as growth factors for tumor cells.
  - The aim is to stop tumor neovascularization.

  - Anti-angiogenesis factors are currently being studied in breast cancer clinical trails.

  - Angiostatin.
    [O'Reilly MS, Cell 79: 315–328, 1994]
    - An angiogenesis inhibitor, which specifically and only inhibits the proliferation of vascular endothelial cells and causes metastases to remain dormant at a microscopic size of (< 0.2 mm).
    - May convert an actively growing tumor into a dormant tumor.

— Endostatin.

— TNP-470.
  — Has demonstrated activity against several human cancers in implanted and nude mice. (breast cancer, glioblastoma, meningioma, neurofibrosarcoma, and prostate cancer).
  — Matrix metalloproteinase inhibitor.
  [Talbot DC, Eur J Cancer 32A: 2528–2533, 1996].
  — Batimastat BB-94.
  — Pre-clinical studies in rats with mammary tumors have demonstrated ↓ incidence of metastases and ↑ survival.
  — Has demonstrated efficacy in phase I studies when used intraperitoneally for malignant ascites and intrapleurally for malignant pleural effusions.

  — Marimastat BB-2516.
  — Carboxyamidotriazole (CAI).
  — Tecogalan sodium.
  — Platelet factor 4.
  — Thalidomide.
  — Tamoxifen.

● HER-2/neu monoclonal antibodies (Herceptin).

[Baselga J, J Clin Oncol 14: 737–744, 1996].
  — Herceptin is a humanized recombinant anti-HER-2/neu monoclonal antibody that targets the HER-2/neu growth factor receptor, inhibiting signal transduction and cell proliferation.

[Cobleigh MA, Proc Am Soc Clin Oncol 17: A376, 1998].
  — Open-label, multinational trial.
  — 222 ♀ with HER-2/neu overexpressing metastatic breast cancer, heavily pretreated, were enrolled.
  — Median follow-up → 11 months.

  — Preliminary RESULTS:
    — Overall response rate → 15%.
      — 6 confirmed CRs.
      — 25 confirmed PRs.
    — Median duration of response → 9.1 months.
    — Median survival → 13 months.

- SIDE EFFECTS of Herceptin:
  - ↓ cardiac ejection fraction observed in 9 patients.
  - 6 of the 9 were symptomatic.
  - All had either prior anthracycline therapy or a significant cardiac history at entry to the trial.
  - One ♀ died of a ventricular arrhythmia.

[Slamon D, Proc Am Soc Clin Oncol 17: A377, 1998].
- Double-blind multinational trial.
- 469 ♀ with metastatic breast cancer, overexpressing HER-2/neu antibody.
- Randomized into four groups:
  - Group 1: 145 ♀ received Adriamycin/cyclophosphamide (AC).
  - Group 2: 146 ♀ received AC + Herceptin.
  - Group 3: 89 ♀ received taxol.
  - Group 4: 89 ♀ received taxol + Herceptin.
- Preliminary RESULTS:
  - ♀ receiving chemotherapy alone had a response rate of 32%.
  - ♀ receiving chemotherapy + Herceptin had a response rate of 49%.
  - Group 1 → 43% response rate.
  - Group 2 → 52% response rate.
  - Group 3 → 16% response rate.
  - Group 4 → 42% response rate.
  - Median follow-up → 10.5 months.
  - Median time to progression:
    - 7.6 months for the chemotherapy + Herceptin group.
    - 4.6 months for the chemotherapy alone group.
  - One year survival.
    - 78% for chemotherapy + Herceptin.
    - 67% for chemotherapy alone.

- SIDE EFFECTS of Herceptin:
  - Myocardial dysfunction was more commonly observed with AC + Herceptin than with AC alone (18 vs. 3%).

- Gemcitabine (Gemzar).
  - Not FDA approved for the treatment of breast cancer.
  - Nucleoside analog.
  - Structurally related to cytarabine (ara-C).

- Once inside the cell, gemcitabine is progressively phosphorylated which then inhibits ribonucleotide reductase and also competes with deoxycytidine triphosphate for incorpation into DNA as a base, hence the DNA chain is terminated.

  [Carmichael J, J Clin Oncol 13: 2731–2736, 1995].
- Phase II study.
- 44 ♀ with locally advanced or metastatic breast cancer.
- 40 ♀ assessable for response.
  - 14 ♀ were chemotherapy-naive.
  - 7 ♀ had received adjuvant chemotherapy.
  - 19 ♀ had received one prior chemotherapy regimen for metastatic disease.
- Gemcitabine was given at a dose of 725 mg/m^2 i.v. over 30 min, once a week, for 3 weeks, followed by a one week rest period every 4 weeks.

- Results:
  - 3 CR's, 7 PR's (overall response rate 25%).
  - Median time to response: 1.9 months.
  - Median survival duration of the 40 ♀: 11.5 months.
- Toxicity:
  - Grade III/IV leukopenia.
  - Nausea/vomiting.
  - Dyspnea.
  - Flu-like symptoms (treatable with acetaminophen).

- Conclusion:
  - Gemcitabine had single-agent activity in metastatic or locally advanced breast cancer.
  - Deserves evaluation in combination chemotherapy.

[Blakstein M, Proc Am Soc Clin Oncol 15: 117 (A135) 1996].
- Phase II study in metastatic breast cancer.
- 36 ♀ enrolled [23 ER(+), nine ER(−), four unknown].
- 31 ♀ postmenopausal, two ♀ perimenopausal, three ♀ premenopausal.
- Median age: 36 years (range 42–85 years old).
- Karnofsky scores had to be > 60 and in most ♀ were ≥ 80.
- None of the ♀ had received chemotherapy for metastatic disease.
- Gemcitabine was given at a dose of 1200 mg/m^2 on days 1, 8 and 15 of a 28 day cycle.

— Results:
  — 2 CR's, ten PR's (overall response rate 46%).
  — 9 stable disease.
  — 5 progressive disease.

— Toxicity:
  — Neutropenia.
  — Nausea/vomiting.
  — Hyperbilirubinemia (1 patient).
  — Cough and pleural effusion (1 patient).
  — Dyspnea (1 patient).

● Capecitabine (Xeloda).
  [Blum JL, Proc Am Soc Clin Oncol 17: A476, 1998].
  — Selectively tumor-activated fluoropyrimidine carbamate.
  — Oral prodrug of 5FU.
  — First metabolism occurs in the liver.
  — Phase II trail in healthy pre-treated ♀.
  — 162 ♀ who had progressed after receiving 2–3 prior chemotherapy regimens.
    — Tumors refractory to anthracycline and taxanes.
  — 62 ♀ premenopausal.
  — 100 ♀ postmenopausal.

  — RESULTS:
    — Response rates:
      — 27 ♀ (20%) out of 135 ♀ with measurable disease.
        — 3 CRs.
        — 24 PRs.
      — 54 ♀ (40%) remained with stable disease.
      — 46 ♀ (34%) had progressive disease.

  — Median duration of response → 241 days.

  — Pain control:
    — 47% of ♀ with pain had a significant response.

- <u>SIDE EFFECTS of Capecitabine:</u>
  - Diarrhea.
  - Hand–foot syndrome.
  - Stomatitis.
  - There is no alopecia or significant myelosuppression.

- Liposomal doxorubicin (Lipodox).
  [Batist G, Cancer Investigation 12(1): 63–64, 1994].
  - Currently in clinical trials in both breast and lung cancer.
  - The hope is it will have less toxicity.

- Amonafide.
  [Ratain MJ, Cancer Investigation 12(1): 38, 1994].
  - Topoisomerase II inhibitor active in leukemia and breast cancer.
  - [CALGB 8862].
    - ♀ with advanced breast cancer.
    - Dose 300 mg/m^2 i.v. over 1 h × 5 days.
    - High correlation between degree of N-acetylation and leukopenia.
    - Optimal dose remains to be determined and may have to be calculated on an individual basis.
  - The investigational new drug permit (IND) has been closed for this drug.
  - This drug is no longer in use.

HIGH-DOSE THERAPY

● High-dose chemotherapy is an investigational approach and its advantage in terms of DFS and/or OS remains to be proven in Randomized trials.

● ~ 7% of breast cancer patients present with stage IV disease.

● ~ 66% of patients with metastatic breast cancer respond to multiagent chemotherapy regimens;
— But only 20% or less achieve a CR.
— At 10 years, < 5% of ♀ with a CR remain disease free.

● The median survival of ♀ diagnosed with metastatic breast cancer is 2 years.

● Factors predicting poor outcome in stage IV patients.
— Exposure to previous adjuvant chemotherapy.
— ≥ 3 organs involved.
— Liver metastases.
— ER(−).

● Bone marrow toxicity is the dose limiting factor for most chemotherapeutic agents
— Poor results with standard chemotherapy doses have led to the study of other treatment alternatives, such as high-dose therapy with bone marrow rescue or peripheral blood progenitor cell (PBPC) rescue.

● The patients most likely to benefit from high-dose therapy are:
— Responders to first induction chemotherapy.
— Patients having received no prior adjuvant chemotherapy.

U.S. Bone marrow transplant regimens

● STAMP 1 BMT regimen (Duke):
— Cyclophosphamide (1875 mg/m^2) over 1 h × 3 days; d(− 6), (− 5), (− 4).
— Cisplatin (55 mg/m^2) c.i. × 3 days; d(− 6), (− 5), (− 4).
— Carmustine (BCNU) (600 mg/m^2) over 2 h × 1 day; day(− 3); after completion of cisplatin.

— Rationale for above regimen:
  — The three drugs interact on DNA at different points, so there is no cross-resistance because they require different mechanisms of repair.
  — Frank Schabel's data supported:
    — There is no cross-resistance between alkylating agents (except thiotepa).
    — There is synergy among alkylating agents.
    — No overlapping side effects.

- STAMP 5 BMT regimen:
  — Cyclophosphamide (1.5 gm/m^2 per day) c.i. × 4 days.
  — Thiotepa (125 mg/m^2 per day) c.i. × 4 days.
  — Carboplatin (200 mg/m^2 per day) c.i. × 4 days.

- Johns Hopkins BMT regimen:
  — Cyclophosphamide (1.5 gm/m^2 per day) c.i. × 4 days.
  — Thiotepa (200 mg/m^2 per day) c.i. × 4 days.

- BUMETH BMT regimen:
  — Busulfan (Myleran) (12 mg/kg) p.o. total dose.
  — Melphalan (100 mg/m^2) over 1 h.
  — Thiotepa (500 mg/m^2) over 1 h.

- Although it appears that high-dose therapy regimens using alkylating agents are efficacious, the best regimen is still unknown.

- Autologous BMT for breast cancer at Duke University:
  [Peters WP, J Clin Oncol 6: 1368–1376, 1988].
  — 60% have CR at 6 weeks and 20% of stage IV patients are disease free at 2 years.
  — 3 of 22 ♀ (14%) premenopausal, HR(−), remained disease free at 8 years.
  — With purges, 50% have CR at 6 weeks and 20% are disease free at 2 years.
  [Jones RB, Cancer 66: 431–436, 1990].

- [Peters WP, Proc Am Soc Clin Oncol 15: (A149) 1996].
  — In the Duke experience, after treatment with AFM chemotherapy (Adriamycin 25 mg/m^2 per d i.v. bolus on days (3), (4), (5); 5FU

750 mg/m^2 per d c.i. on days (1)–(5); and Methotrexate 250 mg/m^2) on day (15) with leucovorin rescue) one-third of patients that result in a PR will go into CR with transplant (conversion rate).

- [Peters WP, New Engl J Med 330: 473–477, 1994].
  – Data from North American transplant centers, in ♀ with metastatic breast cancer receiving induction chemotherapy followed by ABMT as first line therapy, have an overall survival of 35% at 3 years.

- [Bezwoda WR, J Clin Oncol 13: 2483–2489, 1995].
  – Small Randomized study in the metastatic setting.
  – Demonstrated statistically significant survival and DFS in the high-dose arm with marrow rescue when compared to the conventional chemotherapy arm.

- Hematopoietic growth factors have added a new dimension to dose escalation because of their ability to reduce the duration of neutropenia and facilitate early granulocyte recovery. The limitation of this approach remains thrombocytopenia.

- [Peters WP, J Clin Oncol 11: 1132–1143, 1993].
  – Initial data from Duke in collaboration with CALGB has demonstrated, in patients with primary breast cancer with 10 or more (+)LN, an event-free survival of 72% with a median follow-up of 3.3 years and lead follow-up of over 6 years.

- [Peters WP, New Engl J Med 330: 473–477, 1994].
  – Survey of transplant centers in North America requesting primary treatment data on patients treated with ABMT for primary breast cancer.
  – Data was received from 33 institutions.
  – Analyzable information was provided on 662 patients with multinode (+) primary breast cancer.
  – 78% of the patients had 10 or more (+)LN.
  – Three year overall survival for 518 patients with 10 (+)LN was 79% (95% CI: 72–85%) and a three year event-free survival (including all therapy related mortality and relapses) of 71%. (95% CI: 62–79%).
  – Neither tumor size nor high-dose preparative regimens showed statistically significant differences in response rates.

- Patients with HR(+) disease did significantly better than patients who were HR(−).
  - 5-year overall survival: 82% HR(+) patients vs. 70% HR(−) patients. ($P = 0.01$).

- [Antman KH, J Clin Oncol 15(5): 1870–1879, 1997].
  - Data from the Autologous Blood and Transplant Registry of North America (ABMTR).
  - Evaluated 5800 consecutive ♀ in > 130 transplant centers in North America.
  - Between 1989–1995, the number of autotransplants for breast cancer ↑ six times in America.
  - The 100-day mortality ↓ from 22 to 5% ($P < 0.0001$).
  - Substantial ↑ in the use of PBPC's from 14% in 1989 to 70% in 1995.
  - Results of autotransplants correlated with disease stage.
  - Characteristics of ♀ with locally advanced disease (stage II/III):
    - Median age 44 (much younger than average age of ♀ for this stage of disease).
    - Over 70% had > 9 (+) axillary LN's.
  - Characteristics of ♀ with metastatic disease (stage IV):
    - Median age 44 (much younger than average age of ♀ with this stage of disease).
    - 58% of ♀ tumors were ER(+) (Lower percentage than the average ♀ presenting with stage IV disease).
  - 3-year probabilities of progression-free survival.
    - Stage II disease → 65%.
    - Stage III disease → 60%.
    - Stage IV disease.
      - a. If no response to conventional chemotherapy → 7%.
      - b. If partial response to conventional chemotherapy → 13%.
      - c. If complete response to conventional chemotherapy → 32%.

- Recently the use of autologous PBPC's as rescue to the patient s/p high-dose therapy has become more prevalent than rescue with autologous bone marrow transplant.
  - $\sim 2 \times 10^8$ nucleated cells/kg of patient weight consistently results in engraftment.
  - $15–50 \times 10^4$ CFU-GM/kg of patient weight are needed to ensure successful engraftment after myeloblastic chemotherapy.

Ablative protocols used by cancer centers in the USA		
Acronym [reference]	Agent	Dose
STAMP1, CPB [1]	Cyclophosphamide Platinum BCNU	1875 mg/m^2 per day over 1 h $\times$ 3 days 55 mg/m^2 per day c.i. $\times$ 3 days 600 mg/m^2 per day over 2 h $\times$ 1 day
STAMP5, CTCb [2]	Cyclophosphamide Thiotepa Carboplatin	1.5 gm/m^2 per day c.i. $\times$ 4 day 125 mg/m^2 per day c.i. $\times$ 4 days 200 mg/m^2 per day c.i. $\times$ 4 days
CEP [3]	Cyclophosphamide Etoposide Platinum	$1.5–1.75$ gm/m^2 per day $\times$ 3 days $125–200$ mg/m^2 q 12 h $\times$ 6, day 1–3 $40–60$ mg/m^2 per day $\times$ 3 days
Hopkins, CT [4]	Cyclophosphamide Thiotepa	1.5 gm/m^2 per day c.i. $\times$ 4 days 200 mg/m^2 per day c.i. $\times$ 4 days
CT $\pm$ B [5]	Cyclophosphamide Thiotepa $\pm$ BCNU	2.5 gm/m^2 per day $\times$ 3 days 225 mg/m^2 per day $\times$ 3 days 450 mg/m^2
BUMETH [6]	Busulfan Melphalan Thiotepa	12 mg/kg 100 mg/m^2 500 mg/m^2

[1] [Peters WP, J Clin Oncol 6: 1368–1376, 1988].
[2] [Antman KH, J Clin Oncol 10: 102–110, 1992].
[3] [Dunphy FR, J Clin Oncol 8: 1207–1216, 1990].
[4] [Kennedy MJ, J Natl Cancer Inst 83: 920–926, 1991].
[5] [Williams SF, J Clin Oncol 10: 1743–1747, 1992].
[6] [Bensinger WI, Bone Marrow Transplant 19: 1183–1189, 1997].

— The number of PBPCs markedly increases during the recovery phase after myelosuppressive chemotherapy is given.
— $\geq 2 \times 10^6$ CD34$^+$ cells/kg are considered sufficient for a full and timely engraftment.

● Two multicenter prospective Randomized clinical trials in stages II-III with > 10 (+)LN breast cancer patients are underway comparing conventional vs. high-dose therapy.

1. ECOG 2190.
   - Group I: CAF × 6 → Chest wall XRT + tamoxifen, if ER(+).
     Group II: CAF × 6 → High-dose   cyclophosphamide/thiotepa/
       ABMT
       → chest wall XRT and, if ER(+), receive tamoxifen.
       Doses: cyclophosphamide 1.5 gm/m^2 per day c.i. × 4 days
       Thiotepa 200 mg/m^2 per day c.i. × 4 day.

2. CALGB 9082 (The INTERGROUP 0163).
   - Group I: CAF × 4 → standard   cyclophosphamide/platinum/
       BCNU
       → chest wall XRT + tamoxifen, if ER(+).
       Doses: cyclophosphamide 300 mg/m^2 per day × 3 days
       Platinum 30 mg/m^2/ perd × 3 days.
       BCNU 90 mg/m^2 on the 3rd day
   - Group II: CAF × 4 → high-dose   cyclophosphamide/platinum/
       BCNU
       → chest wall XRT + tamoxifen, if ER(+).
       Doses: cyclophosphamide 1875 mg/m^2 per day × days.
       Platinum 55 mg/m^2 per day × 3 days.
       BCNU 600 mg/m^2 on the 3rd day.

High-dose therapy in Europe
[Proc of 20th An Mtg of European Bone Marrow Transplant. Group
(EBMT), Abs 169, 1994].
[Antman K, Bone Marrow Transplantation 10, suppl # 1: 67–73, 1992].

- Over the last years high-dose programs for breast cancer have increased in number.

- In 1997, 2600 ♀ → received high-dose therapy in Europe.

- In 1996, 2136 ♀ → received high-dose therapy in Europe.
  - The vast majority receives PBPC as the only source of hematologic rescue.

- As of July 1998 there were 35 ongoing trials in Europe.
  - 16 of them in the adjuvant setting.
  - The drugs most frequently used are:
    - Cyclophosphamide (72%).

Main ongoing Randomized European Trials in the adjuvant setting				
Group	# LN (+)	Standard arm	High-dose arm	Number of ♀ enrolled to-date
NCI of Milan (Italy)	≥4	Epirubin followed by CMF	HDS	375
Netherlands	≥4	FEC —Epirubicin 120 mg/m²	FEC+CTCb —Epirubicin 120 mg/m²	720
Anglo-Celtic (Cooperative British–Irish group)	≥4	Adriamycin followed by CMF	Adriamycin followed by CT	446
Nordic (Sweden, Norway, Finland)	≥8 or >5*	FEC	FEC+CTCb	500
SFGM/EBMT (French Group)	≥8	FEC	FEC+CAM	286
IBCSG 15–85	≥10 or >5*	EC	High-dose EC	199
German Group	≥10	EC followed by CMF	EC followed by CMT	197

CT   = cyclophosphamide and thiotepa.
CTCb = cyclophosphamide, thiotepa and carboplatin.
FEC   = fluorouracil, epirubicin, cyclophosphamide.
CAM   = cyclophosphamide, melphalan, mitoxantrone.
CMF   = cyclophosphmaide, methotrexate, fluorouracil.
CMT   = cyclophosphamide, mitoxantrone, thiotepa.
EC   = epirubicin, cyclophosphamide.
*   = >5 if bad biological factors [ER(−), high S-phase].
HDS   = high-dose sequential* see following page.

- Carboplatin (65%).
- Thiotepa (48%).
- Melphalan (38%).
- Etoposide (34%).
- Mitoxantrone (21%).
- Ifosfamide (19%).
- No BCNU!

- Similarly to the U.S. trials all receptor positive patients receive tamoxifen.

- A difference with the U.S. trials that remains is the number of positive nodes seen among the patients entering the European Randomized trials.

High dose sequential
Cyclophosphamide 7 gm/m^2 growth factors + apheresis ↓ Methotrexate 8 gm/m^2 + Vincristine 1.4 mg/m^2 ↓ as soon as possible Epirubicin 120 mg/m^2 ↓ every 2–3 weeks Epirubicin 120 mg/m^2 ↓ as soon as possible L-PAM 160–180 gm + Thiotepa 500 mg/m^2 ↓ PBPC

Side effects of high-dose therapy

- Cyclophosphamide.
  - Inactive, must be metabolized.
  - Hemorrhagic myocarditis.
  - Associated with veno-occlusive disease of the liver.
  - Hemorrhagic cystitis.

Main Ongoing Randomized European Trials in the metastatic setting			
Group	When	Standard arm	High-dose arm
EBDIS/EBMT	Upfront	Docetaxel and adriamycin × 3 cycles followed by CMF × 4 cycles	Docetaxel and adriamycin × 3 cycles followed by VIC × 1 cycle, then CT × 1 cycle
Belgian	Upfront	Docetaxel × 4 cycles then AC × 4 cycles	Docetaxel × 3 cycles followed by a 4th cycle of docetaxel with mobilization. Then mitoxantrone-melphalan × 2 cycles (double shot)
SFGM/EBMT	Upfront	FEC × 4 cycles (epirubicin at a dose of 100 mg/m²)	FEC × 4 cycles followed by CT × 1 cycle

EBDIS = European Breast Dose Intensity Study.
EBMT = European Group for Blood and Marrow Transplantation.
SFGM = French Society for Bone Marrow Transplantation.

VIC = etoposide, ifosfamide, carboplatin.
CT = cyclophosphamide and thiotepa.
FEC = fluorouracil, epirubicin, cyclophosphamide.

- Cisplatin.
  - Long half-life.
  - Nephrotoxicity.
  - Ototoxicity.
  - Nausea/vomiting.

- BCNU.
  - Interstitial pneumonitis.
  [Todd NW, Amer Review Respir Disease 147: 1264–1270, 1993].
    - Seen 6 weeks after BMT with peak at 12 weeks by DLCO and clinical symptoms.
    - Usually resolves with steroids.
  - ↓ peripheral vascular resistance, at times requiring vasopressor support.
  - Nausea/vomiting.
  - Hepatotoxicity.

- Hemorrhagic myocarditis.
  [Shabel FM, Cancer Treat Rep 60: 665–698, 1976].
  - Due to high-dose administration of cyclophosphamide.
  - Seen on day(+ 1).
  - Patient complains of fatigue in am → dead by pm.
  - EKG: low voltage → PAC's → PVC's → pump failure.
  - Autopsies reveal blood diffusing among myocytes; however, myocytes are normal.
  - Diagnosed by MRI; blood visible on T_2 images.
  - Therapy:
    - Lots of platelets and supportive care.
    - Thio scavengers used to detoxify alkylating agents.
      - Glutathione.
      - WR2721 (amifostine).
        - SIDE EFFECTS: nausea, vomiting, transient hypotension.
  - Injury is reversible, however must get patient through the next 5–7 days; MUGA eventually returns to normal.
  - Preventable:
    - If give two units of platelets on day(− 2), decreases overall mortality by 3% by avoiding hemorrhagic myocarditis.

- Hemorrhagic cystitis.
  - High-dose cyclophosphamide is associated with a high risk of hemorrhagic cystitis.
  - Reported frequency 6.5–52%.
    - Despite use of hydration protocols.
  - [Lettendre L, Mayo Clin Proc 67: 128–130, 1992].
    - Hyperhydration at 200 ml/m^2 per h during chemotherapy to keep a urinary output at 200 ml/h and continuous bladder irrigation at the rate of 1 l/h, during and for 24 h after high-dose cyclophosphamide, resulted in a very low incidence of microscopic hematuria and no reported cases of visible hematuria.
  - [Meisenberg B, Bone Marrow Transplant 14: 287–291, 1994].
    - 303 evaluable patients, after undergoing high-dose therapy with CPB chemotherapy regimen, outlined above in the Duke protocol.
    - Overall incidence of microscopic hematuria.
      - > 15 rbc/hpf = 19%.
      - > 50 rbc/hpf = 11%.
    - No patient developed visible or symptomatic hematuria.
  - [Shepherd JD, J Clin Oncol 9: 2016–2020, 1991].

— [Hows JM, Br J Cancer 50: 753–756, 1984].
  — Two Randomized trials of prophylaxis with the sulfhydryl-containing compound, Mesna (Mesnex).
  — Have shown mixed results.
  — Were not compared to hyperhydration with continuous bladder irrigation.

● Mucositis.
  — Grade III and IV mucositis may be seen in regimens using melphalan, thiotepa, or VP-16 (etoposide).
  — Possible increased risk of infection.

● Pneumonitis.
  — Infectious.
    — CMV infection [Infections in Medicine, April: 258–262, 1994].
      — Can also cause gastroenteritis, esophagitis, retinitis, hepatitis, fever, leukopenia.
      — Most common cause of infectious death among allogeneic BMT patients with an incidence of 15 and 85% mortality.
      — Occurs ∼ 1–2% of autologous BMT.
      — The greatest risk of developing it is being CMV(+) pre-transplant.
      — Bronchial alveolar lavage is a sensitive and specific diagnostic technique.
      — Therapy:
        — Gancyclovir (Cytovene) + i.v. CMV immune globulin (Cytogan).
                          or
        — Foscarnet (Foscavir) + i.v. CMV immune globulin (Cytogan).
      — Prevention: sero(−) blood products.

  — Chemotherapy induced.
    [Todd NW, Am Rev Respir Dis 147: 1264–1270, 1993].
    — Known offenders.
      — Cyclophosphamide.
      — Carmustine (BCNU).
    — Therapy.
      — Steroids.

- Radiation induced.
- Potentiates drug toxicity with:
  - BCNU.
  - Busulfan.
  - Bleomycin.
  - Mitomycin C.

- Hepatic veno-occlusive disease (VOD).
  - First reported in 1954 in Jamaica among children eating Jamaican bush leaf tea.
  [Bras G, Arch Path 57: 285–300, 1954].
  - 4% incidence, ~ 50% mortality [J Clin Oncol 8: 1699–1706, 1990].
  - Clinical diagnosis.
    - Right upper quadrant pain.
    - Hepatomegaly.
    - Weight gain/ascites.
  - Endothelial damage postulated to be initiating event.
  - No association with gender, hepatitis B serology or preparative regimen.
  [Transplantation 44: 778–783, 1987].
  [Transplantation 39: 603–608, 1985].

  - Prevention.
  [Attal M, Blood 79: 2834–2840, 1992].
    - Prospective, Randomized trial.
    - Heparin 100 U/kg per day c.i. may prevent VOD.

  - Treatment.
    - Supportive.
    - Treat hepatic insufficiency.

- Post transplant hemolytic uremic syndrome (HUS).
  [Juckett M, Bone Marrow Transplant 7: 405–409, 1991].
  - Clinical triad:
    - Microangiopathic hemolytic anemia.
    - Thrombocytopenia.
    - Renal failure.
    - Heterogeneous in presentation and in time course.

- Hepatosplenic candidiasis.
  [Mudad R, Cancer 74(4): 1360–1366, 1994].
  - Clinical presentation.
  - Fever, abdominal pain, ↑ LFTs.
  - Associated with prolonged neutropenia, and older age.
  - Radiologic findings.
  - High attenuation 'target or bulls eye' appearance on CT.
  - Therapy.
  - Amphotericin B and flucytosine.
  - Fluconazole may benefit those who fail amphotericin B.
  - Mortality ~ 35%.

- Low CD4 counts.
  [Peters WP, J Clin Oncol 11(6): 1132–1143, 1993].
  - Patients after transplant have inverted CD4/CD8 ratios for up to 3 years; with about 100 CD4 cell count at 1 year in general; without getting any of the AIDS-related infections, unless exposed to corticosteroids.
  - With corticosteroids, the incidence of pneumocystis carinii pneumonia significantly increases.

- Acute leukemia (AL)/Myelodysplasia (MDS).
  - May develop in patients with completely normal cytogenetic features after high-dose therapy.
  - [Laughlin MJ, J Clin Oncol 16: 1008–1012, 1998].
  - Retrospective review.
  - 864 ♀ with breast cancer who underwent high-dose therapy with CPB chemotherapy regimen and autologous bone marrow support, previously outlined in the Duke regimen above.
  - Five ♀ developed MDS/AL.
  - Pre-transplant cytogenetics on these five ♀ were normal.
  - Post-transplant cytogenetics were abnormal in the four out of five patients tested.
  - The incidence of MDS/AL in this series was relatively low compared to the incidence in patients who undergo autologous bone marrow transplantation for non-Hodgkins lymphoma.

FOLLOWING BREAST CANCER PATIENTS

- Localized disease.
  - Regular P.E. and review of systems with attention to usual metastatic sites (breast, chest wall, lymph nodes, bone, chest, CNS, liver, skin).
  - Regular blood tests (CBC, chemistry profile, LFTs and tumor markers).
    - If LFTs are abnormal, obtain CT scan of the liver.
  - Annual chest X-ray (contraversial; see below ASCO guidelines).
  - Annual mammograms.
  - All ♀ should have pelvic examinations with PAP tests at regular intervals.
  - Bone scan—controversial.

- Current recommendations for mammography after breast cancer treatment.
  - Ipsilateral mammogram 6 months after therapy.
  - Image mastectomy side, if there is remnant tissue.
  - Bilateral mammograms q 1 year.
  - Image of reconstructed breast, at times, is not very informative.
    - Image reconstructed breast at first follow-up to establish a base line, then repeat if clinically indicated.
    - Recurrences are usually superficial and physical examination is more accurate in detecting these lesions.
    - Can create confusion if fat necrosis is present.

- Metastatic disease.
  - Be alert for: impending pathologic fracture, pericardial effusion, pleural effusion, meningeal carcinomatosis, extradural cord compression, hypercalcemia.
  - If LFTs are abnormal.
    - Computerized tomography (CT) scan of the liver.

- Don't forget to assess risk of other family members and recommend screening for them.

- Don't forget to screen for other malignancies such as colorectal, ovarian, cervical and uterine cancers.

- ASCO Guidelines.
  [ASCO Report, J Clin Oncol 15: 2149–2156, 1997].
  - Patients who receive adjuvant therapy require monitoring during therapy, but the value of follow-up of patients after therapy has not been established.
  - Monthly breast self-examination.
  - Annual mammography of the preserved and contralateral breast.
  - Careful history and P.E. every 3–6 months for 3 years, and every 6–12 months for 2 years, then annually.
  - Data are not sufficient to recommend routine bone scans, chest X-rays, hematologic blood counts, tumor markers, liver ultrasonograms or CT scans.
  - All ♀ should have pelvic examinations with PAP tests at regular intervals.

Tumor markers
[Anonymous, J Clin Oncol 14(10): 2843–2877, 1996].

- Non-specific.
  - The data are insufficient to recommend the routine use of tumor markers.
  - In the absence of readily measurable disease they can be used to document treatment failure.

- CA 27.29.
  [Chan DW, J Clin Oncol 15: 2322–2328, 1997].
  - FDA approved.
  - Breast cancer-associated tumor antigen.
  - Controlled prospective clinical trial.
  - 166 ♀ with stage II/III breast cancer.
  - Clinically free of disease after therapy were followed for 2 years.
  - Two consecutive (+) tests yielded a (+) result.
  - Results:
    - Sensitivity 57.7%.
    - Specificity 97.9%.
    - (+) predictive value 92.6%.
  - Conclusion:
    - CA 27.29 was effective in predicting recurrence in patients with both distant and locoregional disease.

- CA 15.3.
  [Hayes DF, J Clin Oncol 4: 1542–1550, 1986].

  — Breast cancer-associated tumor antigen.
  — Enhanced sensitivity in detecting disease progression, but lacks specificity for breast cancer.
  — ↑ in ~75–80% of patients with metastatic disease and ↑ in ~20–50% of patients with newly diagnosed breast cancer.

- Carcinoembryonic antigen (CEA).
  [Hayes DF, J Clin Oncol 4: 1542–1550, 1986].
  — Elevated in 40–50% of the patients with metastatic breast cancer.
  — High levels are particularly indicative of bone or liver mets or multiple sites of disease.
  — Persistently elevated markers post-mastectomy predict increased relapse rates.

- Retrospective study comparing the value of CA 27.29, CA 15.3, and CEA.
  [Mayo JM, Proc Am Soc Clin Oncol 16:(A638), 1997].
  — 126 ♀ with histologic proven breast cancer.
  — 58/126 ♀ (46%) had confirmed metastatic disease.
  — 68/126 ♀ (54%) s/p adjuvant therapy, with no evidence of recurrence.
  — Tumor markers were checked every 3 months over a period of 36 months.
  — Two consecutive (+) tests yielded (+) results.

Results		
Tumor markers	Sensitivity (%)	Specificity (%)
CA 27.29	79	90
CA 15.3	63	89
CEA	54	97

— Conclusion:
  1. CA 27.29 and CA 15.3 had improved sensitivity as compared to CEA.
  2. In this study the lack of tumor marker positivity at the time of recurrent disease correlated with ↓ in DFS, irrespective of ER status.

- CA 549.
  [Chan DW, Am J of Clin Path 101: 465–470, 1994].

% Elevated	5%	14%	32%	74%
Stage	I	II	III	IV

— Lacks specificity.
  — Increased levels occur with other cancers (ovary and liver, etc).
— May be useful with stage IV.

HORMONE REPLACEMENT THERAPY (HRT) IN BREAST CANCER SURVIVORS

[Bluming AZ, Proc Am Soc Clin Oncol 16: (A463), 1997].
[Cobleigh MA, Diseases of the Breast Updates 1(2): 1–10, 1997].
[Colditz GA, Oncology 11(10): 1491–1501, 1997].

- The use of unopposed estrogen after menopause is estimated to ↑ the annual rate of breast cancer risk to 2.1% above that for ♀ not using it. [Pike MC, Epidemiol Rev 15: 17–35, 1993].

- Breast cancer treatment in young ♀ can precipitate premature menopause.

- The standard of care for breast cancer survivors in the USA is to discourage HRT.
  — For fear of activating dormant tumor cells.

- The risk/benefit ratio of administering HRT to breast cancer survivors needs to be determined by a large prospective Randomized trial.
  — There have been a few short term hormone replacement studies done on breast cancer survivors. [Sands R, Menopause 2: 73–80, 1995].
  — HRT for < 2 years does not seem to significantly ↑ the risk of breast cancer recurrence.

- Postmenopausal symptoms include:
  — Hot flashes.
  — Dyspareunia.
  — Atrophic vaginitis.
  — Sleep disturbance.
  — Mood changes.

- Advantages of HRT:
  — HRT alleviates the symptoms listed above.
  — HRT may relieve vasomotor and vaginal symptoms causes by tamoxifen.
  — ↓ incidence of coronary artery disease.
  — ↓ rate of osteoporotic fractures.
  — May ↓ polyps and colon cancer.
  — May protect against Alzheimer's disease.

Menopausal symptoms
[Cobleigh MA, Diseases of the Breast Updates 1(2): 1–10, 1997].

- Hot flashes (vasomotor symptoms).
  - α₂-adrenoreceptor agonists.
  - Clonidine.
    [Goldberg RM, J Clin Oncol 12: 155–158, 1994].
    - Placebo-controlled, double-blind, Randomized clinical trial.
    - Clonidine patches 0.1–0.2 mg/day.
    - Statistically significant ↓ in the frequency of hot flashes.
    - Clonidine patch 44% vs. placebo 27%.
    - SIDE EFFECTS of Clonidine:
      - Constipation.
      - Dry mouth.
      - Drowsiness.
  - Methyldopa.
    [Nesheim BI, Eur J Clin Pharmacol 20: 413–416, 1981].
    - ↓ frequency of hot flashes significantly.
    - Methyldopa 65% vs. placebo 38%.
    - SIDE EFFECTS of Methyldopa:
      - Dry mouth.
      - Tiredness.

  - Vitamin E.
    [Barton DL, J Clin Oncol 16: 495–500, 1998].
    - Placebo-controlled, Randomized, crossover clinical trial.
    - Vitamin E dose of 800 IU daily.
    - 105 ♀ finished the study.
    - Vitamin E does not significantly ↓ hot flashes.
    - Vitamin E 25% vs. placebo 22%.
    - 25% of ♀ may have relief from placebo effect.

  - Dong quai.
    [Hirata JD, Fertil Steril 68(6): 981–986, 1997].
    - Placebo-controlled, double-blind, Randomized clinical trial.
    - 71 postmenopausal ♀ evaluated.
    - Dong quai does not produce estrogen-like responses in endometrial thickness or in vaginal maturation and was no more helpful than placebo in relieving hot flashes.

— Primrose oil.
  — In Wales they have found success with this treatment.
  — It contains linoleic acid which functions as an anti-inflammatory agent, stabilizing adenyl cyclase in the breast.
  — Dose: 2000–3000 mg per day.
  — Randomized clinical trails are needed.

— Megestrol acetate.
  [Loprinzi CL, New Engl J Med 331: 347–352, 1994].
  — Placebo-controlled, double-blind, Randomized clinical trial.
  — Dose: 20 mg p.o. q day.
  — Significantly ↓ frequency of hot flashes.
  — Megace 73% vs. placebo 26%.

— Anticholinergics.
  — Belladonna.
    — Studies need to be done.

— Raloxifene (Evista).
  [Delmas PD, New Engl J Med 337: 1641–1647, 1997].
  — Randomized clinical trial.
  — 601 postmenopausal ♀ evaluated.
  — Raloxifene vs. placebo.
  — Effective and approved for preventing osteoporosis.
  — Can exacerbate hot flashes!

— Medroxyprogesterone acetate.
  [Morrison JC, Am J Obstet Gynecol 138: 99–104, 1980].
  — Placebo-controlled, double-blind, Randomized clinical trial.
  — Single dose of depomedroxyprogesterone acetate 50 mg intramuscular provided relief for 8 weeks.
  — Significantly ↓ frequency of hot flashes.
  — Medroxyprogesterone 68% vs. the placebo 20%.
  — One must be very careful in prescribing progesterone for breast cancer patients because its effect on normal and malignant breast cancer cells is NOT known.

● Vaginal symptoms:
  — Estrogen vaginal cream.
  [Mattsson LA, Acta Obstet Gynecol Scand 62: 393–396, 1983].

- Vaginal estrogen creams, depending on the dose recommended, can raise the serum estrogen level 16–20 times the level with oral administration of the same dose.

— Nonhormonal vaginal lubricant.
[Nachtigall LE, Fertil Steril 61: 178–180, 1994].
- Prospective Randomized open-label trial.
- 15 ♀ evaluated in each treatment group over a 12 week period.
- A nonhormonal local bioadhesive vaginal moisturizer (replens) was a safe and effective alternative to estrogen vaginal cream (premarin).
- Replens did not provide cornification.
- Replens dose: three times per week for at least one month.
- Both exhibited statistically significant ↑ in vaginal, fluid volume, elasticity and a return to the premenopausal pH state.

— One must be very careful in prescribing vaginal estrogen creams to breast cancer patients.

UNUSUAL PRESENTATIONS

Paget disease
[Silverstein MJ, Cancer 77: 2267–2274, 1996].
[Harris JR, Diseases of the Breast, 1996].

- Incidence is ∼ 1–4% of all breast cancers.

- Clinical presentation:
  - Unilateral nipple and areolar change (Fig. 18).
    - Most commonly an eczematoid lesion.
    - Rarely involves the skin of the breast.
  - Serous or serosanguineous discharge may be present, especially in the later stages.
  - Pruritus, burning, and hypersensitivity are common.
  - Almost always accompanied by an underlying malignancy.
    - More commonly DCIS.
    - Invasive ductal carcinoma.

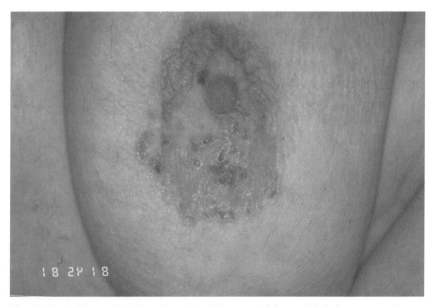

Fig. 18. Paget disease of nipple and areola, without underlying nodule in breast parenchyma.

- The prognosis depends on the presence of an invasive breast cancer and the status of the axillary LNs.

- If no palpable mass is present or mammographic changes suspicious for malignancy, the prognosis is excellent.
  — Breast conservation therapy can be done, always resecting the underlying ductal tissue.

- For patients with an underlying carcinoma, modified radical mastectomy is usually required.
  — The use of systemic therapy follows the same guidelines as for breast cancer.
  — Final results of the EORTC clinical trial should provide valuable information regarding conservative therapy.
  — If breast conservation therapy is done, the nipple areolar complex cannot be preserved due to its involvement.

Breast cancer and pregnancy
[Guinee VF, Lancet; 343: 1587–1589, 1994].
[Petrek JA, Cancer; 67: 869–872, 1991].

- Approximately 1 in 4000 pregnancies is complicated by the appearance of breast cancer.
  — It represents < 3% of all breast cancer cases (pre- and postmenopausal).
  — In childbearing ♀, ∼ 10% of breast cancer cases occur during pregnancy.
- ∼ 70–80% of pregnant ♀ have nodal involvement at diagnosis.

- Prognosis is the same as in age and stage matched non-pregnant patients.

- Clinically suspicious breast masses in pregnant women should be examined via biopsy under local anesthesia.

- Mammography may be difficult to interpret because of pregnancy associated changes of the breast.
  — Ultrasound is often helpful.

- Pregnant patients are candidates for appropriate surgical management under general anesthesia, particularly after the first trimester.

- Radiotherapy is dangerous to the fetus and not a reasonable therapeutic option during any trimester.

- Chemotherapy can be used during the 2nd or the 3rd trimester.
  - A 13% fetal malformation rate was reported among 71 patients receiving chemotherapy during their first trimester.
  - The most common sequelae of chemotherapy given later in the course of pregnancy is low birth weight.
  - Long term effects are unknown.

- Biochemical steroid binding assays for hormone receptors are usually negative.

- Tamoxifen should not be used during pregnancy because of its teratogenic effects.

- Therapeutic abortion has not been shown to improve survival.

Occult breast cancer presenting as solitary axillary mass
[Baron PL, Arch Surg 125: 210–214, 1990].

- First described by Halsted in 1907.

- Axillary masses:
  - 2/3–3/4 of total masses are benign.
  - 1/3–1/4 are malignant.
  - Most commonly, lymphoma, breast, lung, and melanoma.

  - Could be due to small foci of breast tissue in the axilla.

- Mammograms may be (−).

- Overall survival does not differ greatly in these ♀ from other ♀ with the same amount of LN involvement with a known primary.

- These ♀ should be treated like any other stage II breast cancer patient, including chemotherapy.

- Most ♀ to-date have received mastectomy as the surgical approach.

- MRI may be useful.

Phyllodes tumor (Fig. 19)
[Rowell MD, Am J Surg 165: 376–379, 1993].
[Christensen L, Eur J Cancer 29A(13):1824–31 1993].

- Old name: Cystosarcoma phylloides.

- Definition:
  - Rare fibroepithelial breast tumor, typically presenting in the fourth decade.

- Clinical manifestations:
  - Can present in a wide spectrum, ranging from benign to malignant lesions with metastases.
  - Usually bulky, painless, multinodular breast mass.
    - May grow rapidly causing increased pressure in the skin leading to varicose veins, shiny stretched skin and even ulcerations over a massive tumor.
    - The skin is not involved.

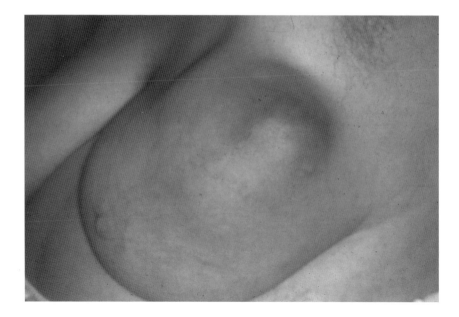

Fig. 19. Large-size phyllode tumor. Notwithstanding the benign nature of this lesion, mastectomy is sometimes necessary to avoid the possibility of non-benign local recurrence.

— Increase in size of ipsilateral LN may be seen in ~ 20% of the patients, however this increase usually is not due to metastases.

- On mammography and ultrasound: very similar to fibroadenoma.

- Pathology:
  — Well-circumscribed.
  — Lacks a true capsule.
  — The stroma determines whether it is benign or malignant.
  — Leaf-like projections and stromal cellularity differentiate it from fibroadenoma.
  — Histologic distinction between benign and malignant phyllodes is very difficult at times, therefore there is a 'borderline' phyllodes tumor.

- Recurs locally in ~ 20% of the patients with incomplete excision.

- Most common site of distant metastases, in order:
  — Lungs.
  — Bones.
  — Liver.
  — Lymph nodes.

- Treatment:
  — Requires complete extirpation with a wide margin of normal tissue.
  — There is no biologic rationale for routine mastectomy, since these tumors are not multicentric.
  — Axillary dissection is not indicated.
  — The use of adjuvant therapy should follow guidelines for sarcoma and not breast cancer.
    — Ifosfamide and adriamycin seem to be the most active agents for metastatic disease.
  — The role of hormonal manipulation is still not known.

MALE BREAST

[Gately CA. Male Breast Disease. The Breast 7: 121–127, 1998].
- Sclerosing adenosis.
  - Reported in association with small cell carcinoma of the lung.

- Phyllodes tumor.
  - Reported in association with gynecomastia secondary to prolonged estrogen therapy for prostate carcinoma.

Male Breast Cancer

[Lipshy K, Contemporary Surgery 49(2): 71–75, 1996].
[Adami HO, Cancer 64(6): 1177–1182, 1989].

- Epidemiology:
  - ~ 1000 cases diagnosed in the US per year.
  - incidence among US blacks.
  - In the UK 0.7% of all breast cancer.
  - Mean age of male breast cancer in the US is ~ 60 years of age.
  - In parts of sub-Saharan Africa, ~ 3–10% of all breast cancer occurs among males.

- Risk factors:
  - Male electrical line workers are at an ↑ risk.
  - Ionizing radiation and electromagnetic fields have been implicated.
  - Does not appear to be in association with gynecomastia.
  - May have inherited component, mechanisms are unknown.
    - Lifetime risk for a male with an affected mother and sister is 2.3%.
  - Does not appear to be linked to BRCA1.
  - ↑ in BRCA2 gene mutation families.
  - Germline mutations in the androgen receptor (chromosome Xq11.2-12) have been observed. [Lobaccaro JM, Hum Mol Genet 2: 1799–1802, 1993]
  - Klinefelter's syndrome (XXY) → 66.5 × risk of general population.
    - Non-disjunction leads to the chromosome abnormality of an XXY male.
    - Characteristics of Klinefelter's syndrome.
      - Phenotypically ♂.
      - Eunuchoid habitus.

- 2° sexual characteristics at puberty do not fully develop.
- Female hair distribution.
- Gynecomastia (40%).
- Short stature.
- Hypogonadism (testicular atrophy).
- Infertility.
- Plasma testosterone levels average $\sim$ half of normal.
- $\uparrow$ FSH and $\uparrow$ LH.

- Pathology:
  - Almost always infiltrating ductal carcinoma.
  - Lobular histology seen only in cases of hyper-estrogenism such as in Klinefelter's syndrome. However, all other variants of breast cancer also occur including Pagets disease.

- Clinical presentations:
  - In UK the mean age of presentation is 64 years of age.
  - The left breast is affected more than the right.
  - The disease generally parallels the condition in ♀, but tends to present in an older age and in a more advanced stage.
  - Skin and chest fixation are more frequent than in ♀.
  - 90% present with breast lump.
    - Painless mass.
  - 20% present with nipple changes.
  - 14% present with nipple discharge.
  - 4% have breast pain at presentation.
  - 3% present with metastatic disease.
  - Asymmetry, eccentricity, firmness, fixation, or ulceration of the breast should raise suspicion.
  - Mammography.
    - Is useful.
    - Same sensitivity in ♂ and ♀.
    - Ultrasound may also be useful.

- Therapy:
  - Multidisciplinary.
  - Due to its usual central location, modified radical mastectomy with LN dissection followed by XRT to the chest wall is the usual treatment of choice.

- Adjuvant chemotherapy and/or endocrine therapy are used with an aim to improve survival.
- Great propensity for local recurrence, so treat extensively.
- Likely to be ER(+); most patients respond well to endocrine therapy such as tamoxifen, progesterone and orchiectomy.
- Adjuvant chemotherapy has been used for LN(+) primary disease and that benefits seem similar to those seen in ♀.
  - If 10 (+)LN → only 10% of the patients will be disease free (DF) in 10 years.
  - If 4–9 (+)LNs → 25% will be DF in 10 years.
  - If 1–3 (+)LNs → 50% will be DF in 10 years.
  - If no nodes are involved → 70% will be DF in 10 years.

- Prognosis:
  - Axillary LN involvement is the #1 prognostic factor.
  - LN(−) patients with primary tumors > 2 cm experience a risk of relapse more than twice as great as those with lesions < 1 cm.
  - Believed to be worse than in ♀.

CHEMOPREVENTION

[Veronesi U, 15th Annual International Miami Breast Cancer Conference. February 26–28, 1998].

[Powles TJ, Oncology 12(3 suppl 5): 28–31, 1998].

Tamoxifen chemoprevention trials

- ∼ 20 000 ♀ without breast cancer are involved in longterm Randomized trials worldwide.

- Breast Cancer Prevention Trial (BCPT).
  NSABP-P1
  − 13 388 ♀ enrolled.
  − Double-blind, placebo-controlled, Randomized trial, launched in April 1992.
  − Healthy ♀ at risk of developing breast cancer.
    − ♀ 35–59 years of age had to have a family history which ↑ their risk to that of a 60-year-old ♀.
    − ♀ > 59 years of age did not have to be at special risk.
  − African American ♀, Asian American, Hispanic, and other groups together made up ∼ 3% of the participants.

Initial Results of NSABP and NCI Trial (BCPT) April 1992–September 1997		
	Number of women affected in the tamoxifen Group	Number of ♀ affected in the placebo Group
Invasive breast cancer	85	154
Breast cancer deaths	3	5
DCIS	31	59
Endometrial carcinoma	33	14
Pulmonary embolism	17	6
Deep venous thrombosis	30	19
Bone fractures of hip, wrist, and spine	47	71
Heart attacks	No difference in the treatment groups	

- ♀ Randomized to tamoxifen 20 mg/day vs. placebo.
- This trial closed in September of 1997.
- Initial results:
  - Shows a 45% reduction in breast cancer incidence among the healthy but high-risk for breast cancer ♀ who took tamoxifen.
- On March 24, 1998, the study committee recommended that the participants and their physicians be told what pills each participant had been taking because of the clear evidence that tamoxifen reduced breast cancer.

- Italian trial.
  [Veronesi U, Lancet 352: 93–97, 1998].
  - National Cancer Institute in Milan.
  - Double-blind, placebo-controlled, Randomized trial.
  - Healthy ♀, > 45 years of age who were not at ↑ risk of developing breast cancer, and who had undergone hysterectomy, were enrolled.
  - ♀ Randomized to tamoxifen 20 mg p.o./day vs. placebo × 5 years.
  - 5408 ♀ enrolled.
    - 2708 ♀ in placebo arm.
    - 2700 ♀ in the tamoxifen arm.
  - Mean age is 51 years.
  - Median follow-up is 46 months.

  - Preliminary results:
    - No statistical significance between arms.
    - 41 cases of breast cancer have occurred.
      - Tamoxifen arm → 19 cases.
      - Placebo arm → 22 cases.
    - No deaths from breast cancer.
    - There was a statistically significant reduction of breast cancer among ♀ receiving tamoxifen who also used hormone replacement therapy (HRT) during the trial.
      - Out of 390 ♀ on HRT + placebo → eight cases of breast cancer.
      - Out of 362 ♀ on HRT + tamoxifen → 1 case of breast cancer.
    - There was a statistically significant ↑ risk of vascular events in the tamoxifen arm.
      - 18 ♀ on placebo.
      - 38 ♀ on tamoxifen ($P = 0.0053$).

  - Conclusion:
    - Preliminary analysis.

- The postulated protective effects of tamoxifen are not yet apparent.
- ♀ using HRT appear to have benefitted from using concurrent tamoxifen.

● International Breast Cancer Intervention Study (IBIS).
  - UK.
  - Recruiting began in 1992.
  - Healthy ♀, aged 40–65 years of age, who had at least a 2-fold ↑ risk of subsequently developing breast cancer, were enrolled.
  - ♀ Randomized to tamoxifen p.o. 20 mg/day vs. placebo.
  - > 4000 ♀ enrolled to-date.

● Royal Marsden Hospital Tamoxifen Chemoprevention Trial.
  [Powles TJ, J Clin Oncol 14: 78–84, 1996].
  - Randomized controlled tamoxifen chemoprevention trial among healthy ♀.
  - 2500 healthy ♀ randomized:
    - Placebo p.o./day × 8 years
            vs.
    - Tamoxifen 20 mg p.o./day × 8 years.

Raloxifene chemoprevention trials

● Raloxifene (Evista).
  [Delmas P, New Engl J Med 337(23): 1641–1647, 1997].
  - Like tamoxifen
    - It is a selective estrogen receptor modulator (SERM).
    - ↑ bone mineral density in postmenopausal ♀.
    - ↓ serum cholesterol.
  - It has no known estrogenic effect on the endometrium.
  - FDA approved raloxifene for use in decreasing fracture rate in ♀ at risk of osteoporosis.
  - Current osteoporosis trials have more than 14000 healthy post-menopausal ♀ at no special risk of developing breast cancer on raloxifene.
    - ♀ in these trials are having annual mammography.
    - These trials should identify any chemoprevention effect of raloxifene.

● Multiple outcomes of Raloxifene.
  [Proc Am Soc Clin Oncol 17: A3, 1998].

— Post-menopausal ♀ with osteoporosis who took Raloxifene for 2 1/2 years to prevent fractures had a significant 70% ↓ in breast cancer risk.
— 7704 osteoporotic ♀, < 80 years of age.
— ♀ had no prior history of breast or endometrial cancer.
— Mean age of ♀ was 66.5 years.
— Randomized to placebo vs. Raloxifene 60 or 120 mg per day.
— Median follow-up → 33 months.
— Trial will continue in Randomized fashion × 5 more years.
— Preliminary RESULTS:
  — Invasive breast cancer.
    — 13 cases in Raloxifene group vs. 22 cases in placebo group ($P < 0.001$).
    — The risk reduction in breast cancer was similar in ♀ receiving either 60 or 120 mg/day of Raloxifene.

  — Endometrial cancer.
    — 4 cases in Raloxifene group vs. 4 cases in placebo group.
  — Venous thrombosis and pulmonary emboli.
    — The risk with Raloxifene is similar to that of Tamoxifen and Estrogen.

● The study of Tamoxifen and Raloxifene (STAR).
  — NSABP double-blind Randomized trial.
  — Scheduled to begin at the end of 1998.
  — 22 000 postmenopausal ♀, 35 years of age or older, at high risk for breast cancer, will be Randomized to 5 years of Tamoxifen 20 mg p.o./day vs. 5 years of Raloxifene 60 mg p.o./day.

Retinoids chemoprevention trials

Proposed as cancer chemoprevention agents due to their differentiating properties.

● Isotretinoin
  — ↓ occurrence of second primary tumors in patients previously treated for squamous cell carcinoma of the head and neck.
  — One-third of the patients receiving isotretinoin did not complete the 12 month course of treatment because of toxicity or noncompliance.

- Fenretide (4-HPR).
  - Synthetic retinoid.
  - Preferential accumulation of the compound in the breast instead of the liver.
  - 1984 4-HPR Randomized trial in breast cancer patients found prohibitive toxicity.
    - Toxicity was encountered at 600 mg/day and 800 mg/day.
      - Night blindness.
      - Erythema.
  - 1986 4-HPR trial identified the best tolerable dose at 200 mg/day with a 3 day treatment interruption at the end of each month.
  - 4-HRP Randomized trial.
    - 2972 enrolled from 3/87 to 7/93.
    - ♀ age 30–70 with LN(−) breast cancer and T_1 or T_2 < 5 cm.
    - All ♀ received radical surgery or conservative surgery with XRT.
    - 2849 evaluable ♀.
      - 1422 ♀ in the 4-HPR group.
      - 1427 in the control group.
    - 1910 ♀ have completed the first 5 years.
    - 840 ♀ have interrupted the study.
    - Results will be available in 2 years.

Index

Breast Cancer:

A Guide for Fellows

Appendix 1
Complete Citations

Orlando E. Silva, M.D.
Stefano Zurrida, M.D.

1999

Presented by Umberto Veronesi, M.D.

Books

AMERICAN JOINT COMMITTEE FOR CANCER STAGING AND END RESULTS, Lippincott-Raven, 1983.

AMERICAN JOINT COMMITTEE ON CANCER (AJCC) CANCER STAGING MANUAL, ID Fleming (Ed) Lippincott-Raven, pp. 171–180, 1997.

BREAST IMAGING, Kopans DB. Philadelphia, JB Lippincott, 1998.

DISEASES OF THE BREAST. Edited by: JR Harris, ME Lippman, M Morrow, and S Hellman. Lippincott-Raven Publishers, Philadelphia, 1996.

DUCTAL CARCINOMA IN SITU OF THE BREAST. Silverstein MJ (ed). Williams and Wilkins, Baltimore, 1997.

HANDBOOK FOR STAGING OF CANCER. Manual for Staging of Cancer, 1st Edition, 1998. Lippincott-Raven.

PATHOLOGY OF THE BREAST. Tavassoli FA. Elsevier 1992.

Book chapters

Hortobagyi GN, Buzdar AU, Locally advanced breast cancer: A review including the MD Anderson Experience. IN: HIGH RISK BREAST CANCER. Ragaz J, Ariel IM (eds) Berlin. Springer, 1991 pp. 382–415.

Silverstein MJ, Van Nuys ductal carcinoma in situ classification. IN: DUCTAL CARCINOMA IN SITU OF THE BREAST. Silverstein MJ (editor) Williams and Wilkins, Baltimore, pp. 247–257.

Conferences

3rd International Conference on Adjuvant Therapy of Breast Cancer; March 2–5, 1988, St. Gallen, Switzerland.

Palm Beach Breast Cancer Conference: An International Symposium, February 17–19, 1994.

12th Annual International Breast Cancer Conference, March 16–18, 1995. Swain SM, Chemotherapy: toxicities of adjuvant therapy and high dose therapy with autologous bone marrow transplant (Meeting abstract).

15th Annual International Miami Breast Cancer Conference. February 26–28, 1998.
Presentations by: Blamey RW, Fowble B, Kopans DB, Veronesi U.

20th Annual San Antonio Breast Cancer Symposium. Dec 3–6, 1997. Abstracts/Presentations:

— Comparison of overall survival in two trials comparing letrozole 25 mg, Femara) with megestrol acetate or with aminoglutethimide in patients with advanced breast cancer. Smith IE, Chaudri HA, Lassus M, Hornberger U.

— The natural history of breast cancer: What have we learned from screening? 16-year year follow-up of 2500 women, mortality and survival data, tumor progression, therapeutic implications. Tabar L.

— The effect of increasing dose-intensity and cummulative dose of adjuvant cyclophosphamide in node (+) breast cancer: Results of NSABP-B25. Wolmark N, Fisher B, Anderson S.

Articles (Alphabetical and chronological order by publication).

Acta Cytol 31: 301–4, 1987. The value of routine cytologic examination of breast cyst fluids. Ciato S, Cariaggi P, Bulgaresi P.

Acta Obstet Gynecol Scand 62(5): 393–396, 1983. Vaginal absorption of two estriol preparations A comparative study in postmenopausal women. Mattsson LA, Cullberg G.

Acta Oncol 27: 483–487, 1988. Importance of tumor cells in axillary node sinus margins, (clandestine metastases) discovered by serial sectioning in operable breast carcinoma. Friedman S, Bertin F, Mouriesse H, Benchabat A, Genin J, Sarrazin D, Contesso G.

Adjuvant Therapy of Cancer, 5: 347, 1987. Southeastern Cancer Study Group (SEG).

Adv Surg 30: 209–221, 1996. The role of the sentinel lymph node in the management of patients with breast cancer. Statman R, Giuliano AE.

Arch Path 57: 285–300, 1954. Veno-occlusive disease, VOD) of the liver with nonportal type of cirrhosis, occuring in Jamaica [First reported in 1954 in Jamaica among children eating Jamaican bush leaf tea] Bras G, Jelliffe DB, Stuart KL.

Arch Surg 125: 210–214, 1990. Occult breast cancer presenting with axillary metastases Updated management. Baron PL, Moore MP, Kinne DW, Candela FC, Osborne MP, Petrek JA.

Am J Clin Oncol 12: 453–455, 1989. Continuous intravenous infusion of 5-fluorouracil in the treatment of refractory breast cancer. Chang AY, Most C, Pandya KJ.

Am J Clin Oncol 14: 60–65, 1991. Local-regional recurrences of breast cancer: treatment with radiation therapy and local microwave hyperthermia. Amichetti M, Valdagni R, Graiff C, Valentini A.

Am J Clin Oncol 14: 30–32, 1991. 5-Fluorouracil plus leucovorin in women with metastatic breast cancer A phase II study. Loprinzi CL, Ingle JN, Schaid DJ, Buckner JC, Edmonson JH, Allegra CJ.

Am J Clin Oncol 19: 451–454, 1996. Karasek K, Deutsch M. Lumpectomy and breast irradiation for breast cancer after radiotherapy for lymphoma.

Am J Clin Oncol 20(5): 493–9, 1997. Induction intra-arterial chemotherapy for T4 breast cancer through an implantable port-catheter system. Chang HT, Mok KT, Tzeng WS.

Am J Clin Pathol 101: 465–70, 1994. Breast cancer marker Ca549 A multicenter study. Chan DW, Beveridge RA, Bhargava A, Wilcox PM, Kennedy MJ, Schwartz MK.

Am J Epidemiol 135: 190–199, 1992. The Li-Fraumeni syndrome: from clinical epidemiology to molecular genetics. Strong LC, Williams WR, Tainsky MA.

Am J Epidemiol 143: 543–552, 1996. Breast cancer and lactation history in Mexican women. Romieu I, Hernandez-Avila M, Lazcano E, Lopez L, Romero-Jaime R.

Am J Med 92: 539–548, 1992. Prognostic indicators in node-negative early stage breast cancer. Wong WW, Vijayakumar S, Weichselbaum RR.

Am J Pathol 147: 9–19, 1995. Intratumor microvessel density as a prognostic factor in cancer. Weidner N.

Am J Surg 165: 376–379, 1993. Phyllodes tumors. Rowell MD, Perry RR, Hsiu JG, Barranco SC.

Am J Surg Pathol 2: 39–46, 1978. Relationship of necrosis and tumor border to lymph node metastases and 10-year survival in carcinoma of the breast. Carter D, Pipkin RD, Shepard RH, Elkins RC, Abbey H.

Am Rev Respir Dis 147: 1264–1270, 1993. Pulmonary drug toxicity in patients with primary breast cancer treated with high-dose combination chemotherapy and autologous bone marrow transplantation. Todd NW, Peters WP, Ost AH, Roggli VL, Piantadosi CA.

Ann Intern Med 58: 136–142, 1963. Cowden's disease: a possible new symptom complex with multiple system involvement. Lloyd KM, Dennis M.

Ann Intern Med 71: 747–752, 1969. Soft tissue sarcomas, breast cancer, and other neoplasms: a familial syndrome? Li FP, Fraumeni JF jr.

Ann Intern Med 108: 345–349, 1988. Pleural fluid pH in malignant effusions Diagnostic, prognostic, and therapeutic implications. Sahn SA, Good JT.

Ann Intern Med 115: 401–403, 1991. The optimal timing of mastectomy: low tide or high tide? McGuire WL.

Ann Intern Med 119: 655–660, 1993. Medical hazards of obesity. Pi-Sunyer FX.

Ann Intern Med 120: 18–25, 1994. Obesity as an adverse prognostic factor for patients receiving adjuvant chemotherapy for breast cancer. J Bastarrachea, Hortobagyi GN, Smith TL, Kau SW, Buzdar AU.

Ann Intern Med 124: 897–905, 1996. Breast cancer in black women. Moormeier J.

Ann Intern Med 128(2): 114–117, 1998. Radiation therapy for breast cancer and increased risk for esophageal carcinoma. Ahsan H, Neugut AI.

Ann Med 29(1): 31–35, 1997. Radioisotopes in the treatment of bone metastases. Ben-Josef E, Porter AT.

Ann Oncol 2: 347–354, 1991. Effects of primary chemotherapy in conservative treatment of breast cancer patients with operable tumors larger than 3 cm: Results of a randomized trial in a single centre. Mauriac L, Durand M, Avril A, Dilhuydy JM.

Ann Plast Surg 32(3): 234–241, March 1994. The free transverse rectus abdominis musculocutaneous flap for breast reconstruction: one center's experience with 211 consecutive cases. Schusterman MA, Kroll SS, Miller MJ, Reece GP, Baldwin BJ, Robb GL, Altmyer CS, Ames FC, Singletary SE, Ross MI, et al.

Ann Surg 20: 497–555, 1894. The results of operations fo the cure of cancer of the breast performed at The Johns Hopkins Hospital from June 1889 to January 1894. Halsted WS.

Ann Surg 194: 585–591, 1981. Axillary micro- and macrometastases in breast cancer: prognostic significance of tumor size. Rosen PP, Saigo PE, Braun DW, Weathers E, Fracchia AA, Kinne DW.

Ann Surg 197: 276–283, 1983. Discontinuous or ski" metastases in breast carcinoma Analysis of 1228 axillary dissections. Rosen PP, Lesser ML, Kinne DW, Beattie EJ.

Ann Surg 220: 391–398, 1994. Lymphatic mapping and sentinel lymphadenectomy for breast cancer. Giuliano AE, Kirgan DM, Guenther JM, Morton DL.

Ann Surg 222(5): 612–618, November 1995. Conservation surgery after primary chemotherapy in large carcinomas of the breast. Veronesi U, Bonadonna G, Zurrida S, Galimberti V, Greco M, Brambilla C, Luini A, Andreola S, Rilke F, Raselli R, Merson M, Sacchini V, Agresti R.

Ann Surg 226(3): 271–276, 1997. Histopathologic validation of the sentinel lymph node hypothesis for breast carcinoma Turner RR, Ollila DW, Krasne DL, Giuliano AE.

Ann Surg Oncol 2: 207–213, 1995. Treatment trends for ductal carcinoma in situ of the breast. Winchester DP, Menck HR, Osteen RT, Kraybill W.

Ann Surg Oncol; 3(1): 57–61, 1996. Interpretation of the risk associated with the unexpected finding of lobular carcinoma in situ. Zurrida S, Bartoli C, Galimberti V, Raselli R, Barletta L.

Ann Thorac Surg 54: 244–247, 1992. Long-term survival after resection of pulmonary metastases from carcinoma of the breast. Lanza LA, Natarajan G, Roth JA, Putnam JB.

Anticancer Drugs 7: 9–12, 1996. First-line treatment of metastatic breast cancer. Trudeau ME.

Anticancer Res 16: 3913–3917, 1996. Axillary dissection can be avoided in selected breast cancer patients: analysis of 401 cases. Greco M, Agresti R, Raselli R, Giovanazzi R, Veronesi U.

Arch Surg 116: 748–751, 1981. Staging of breast cancer: a new rationale for internal mammary node biopsy. Morrow M, Foster RS.

Arch Surg 122: 1244–1247, 1987. The significance of local control in the primary treatment of breast cancer Lucy Wortham James clinical research award. Hayward J, Caleffi M.

Arch Surg 124: 21–25, 1989. The prognostic significance of lymph node metastases after preoperative chemotherapy for locally advanced breast cancer. McCready DR, Hortobagyi GN, Kau SW, Smith TL, Buzdar AU, Balch CM.

Arch Surg 127: 1392–1395, 1992. Ten year follow-up of breast carcinoma in situ in Connecticut. Ward BA, McKhann CF, Ravikkumar TS.

Biology of Blood and Marrow Transplantation 3: 91–97, 1997. The significance of tumor contamination in the bone marrow from high-risk primary breast cancer patients treated with high-dose chemotherapy and hematopoietic support. Vredenburgh JJ, Silva O, Broadwater G, Berry D, DeSombre K, Tyer C, Petros WP, Peters WP, Bast RC.

Blood 79: 2834–2840, 1992. Prevention of hepatic veno-occlusive disease after bone marrow transplant by continuous infusion of low dose heparin: a prospective randomized trial. Attal M, Huguet F, Rubie H.

Bone Marrow Transplant 7: 405–409, 1991. Hemolytic uremic syndrome following bone marrow transplantation. Juckett M, Perry EH, Daniels BS, Weisdorf DJ.

Bone Marrow Transplant 10 Suppl 1: 67–73, 1992. Dose intensive therapy in breast cancer. Antman K, Corringham R, de Vries E, Elfenbein G, Gianni AM, Gisselbrecht C, Herzig R, Juttner C, Kaizer H, Kennedy MJ, et al.

Bone Marrow Transplant 14: 287–291, 1994. Prevention of hemorrhagic cystitis after high-dose alkylating agent chemotherapy and autologous bone marrow support. Meisenberg B, Lassiter M, Hussein A, Ross M, Vredenburgh JJ, Peters WP.

Bone Marrow Transplant; 19(12): 1183–9, 1997. High-dose busulfan, melphalan, thiotepa and peripheral blood stem cell infusion for the treatment of metastatic breast cancer. Bensinger WI, Schiffman KS, Holmberg L, Appelbaum FR, Maziarz R, Montgomery P, Ellis E, Rivkin S, Weiden P, Lilleby K, Rowley S, Petersdorf S, Klarnet JP, Nichols W, Hertler A, McCroskey R, Weaver CH, Buckner CD.

The Breast 7: 121–127, 1998. Gately CA. Male Breast Disease.

The Breast 7: 150–153, 1998. Laparoscopic oophorectomy: an emerging option for the management of breast cancer. Walsh D, Humeniuk V, Parkyn R.

Breast Disease 7: 353–360, 1994. Ductal carcinoma in situ of the breast: Comedo versus non Comedo subtype non predictors of recurrence or contralateral new breast primary. Archher SG, Kemp BL, Gadd M, Shallenberger R, Ames FC, Singletary SE.

Br J Cancer 11: 359–377, 1957. Histological grading and prognosis in breast cancer:, A study of 1409 cases of which 359 were followed for 15 years. Bloom HJG, Richardson WW.

Br J Cancer 50: 231–233, 1984. Decreased natural killer cell activity and interferon production by leucocytes in patients with adenocarcinoma of the pancreas. Funa K, Nilsson B, Jacobsson G, Alm GV.

Br J Cancer 50: 753–756, 1984. Comparison of Mesna with forced diuresis to prevent cyclophosphamide-induced hemorrhagic cystitis in bone marrow transplant A Prospective Randomized study. Hows JM, Mehta A, Ward L, et al.

Br J Cancer 53: 629–636, 1986. The use of an LH-RH agonist, ICI 118630, Zoladex) in advanced premenopausal breast cancer. MR Williams, Walker KJ, Turkes A, Blamey RW, Nicholson RI.

Br J Cancer 63: 447–450, 1991. The long term prognostic significance of c-erbB-2 in primary breast cancer. Winstanley J, Cooke T, Murray GD, Platt-Higgins A, George WD, Holt S, Myskov M, Spedding A, Barraclough BR, Rudland PS.

Br J Cancer 66: 523–527, 1992. Prognostic significance of breast cancer axillary lymph node micrometastases assessed by two special techniques: reevaluation with longer follow-up. Mascarel de, Bonichon, F, Coindre JM, Trojani M.

Br J Cancer 68(5): 969–973, 1993. Spinal cord compression in breast cancer: a review of 70 cases. Hill ME, Richards MA, Gregory WM, Smith P, Rubens RD.

Br J Cancer 74: 297–299, 1996. Randomised comparison of 5 years of adjuvant tamoxifen with continuous therapy for operable breast cancer: The Scottish Cancer Trials Breast Group. Stewart HJ, Forrest AP, Everington D, McDonald CC, Dewar JA, Hawkins RA, Prescott RJ, George WD.

Br J Cancer; 74(11): 1838–42, 1996. Mammographic screening after the age of 65 years: early outcomes in the Nijmegen programme. van Dijck J, Verbeek A, Hendriks J, Holland R, Mravunac M.

Br J Cancer 75(4): 602–605, 1997. Clodronate improves bone mineral density in post-menopausal breast cancer patients treated with adjuvant antioestrogens. Saarto T, Blomqvist C, Valimaki M, Makela P, Sarna S, Elomaa I.

Br J Cancer 75: 1318–1323, 1997. Early-onset breast cancer: histopathologic and prognostic considerations. Kollias J, Elston CE, Ellis IO, Robertson JFR, Blamey RW.

Br J Cancer 76(2): 270–277, 1997. Comparison of toremifene and tamoxifen in post-menopausal patients with advanced breast cancer: a randomized double-blind, the nordic phase III study. Pyrhonen S, Valavaara R, Modig H, Pawlicki M, Pienkowski T, Gundersen S, Bauer J, Westman G, Lundgren S, Blanco G, Mella O, Nilsson I, Hietanen T, Hindy I, Vuorinen J, Hajba A.

Br J Plast Surg 47(7): 495–501, October 1994. Refinements in free flap breast reconstruction: the free bilateral deep inferior epigastric perforator flap anastomosed to the internal mammary artery. Blondeel PN, Boeckx WD.

Br J Plast Surg 50(5): 315–321, July 1997. The fate of the oblique abdominal muscles after free TRAM flap surgery. Blondeel N, Boeckx WD, Vanderstraeten GG, Lysens R, Van Landuyt K, Tonnard P, Monstrey SJ, Matton G.

Br J Plast Surg 50(5): 322–330, July 1997. The donor site morbidity of free DIEP flaps and free TRAM flaps for breast reconstruction. Blondeel N, Vanderstraeten GG, Monstrey SJ, Van Landuyt K, Tonnard P, Lysens R, Boeckx WD, Matton G.

Br J Surg 46: 574–582, 1959. The lymphatics of the breast. RT Turner-Warwick.

Br J Surg 54: 191–195, 1967. Multiple primary carcinomata of the colon, duodenum, and larynx associated with kerato-acanthomata of the face. Muir EG, Bell AJ, Barlow KA.

Br J Surg 70: 60–63, 1983. Dixon JM, Anderson TJ, Lumsden AB, Elton RA, Roberts MM, Forrest APM. Mammary duct ectasia.

Br J Surg 76(2): 185–186, February 1989. Residual tumour after biopsy for non-palpable ductal carcinoma in situ of the breast. Wobbes T, Tinnemans JG, van der Sluis RF.

Br J Surg 83(6): 820–822, June 1996. Periductal mastitis and duct ectasia: different conditions with different aetiologies. Dixon JM, Ravisekar O, Chetty U, Anderson TJ.

Br Med J 2: 643–647, 1937. Conservative treatment of cancer of the breast. Keynes G.

Br Med J 297(6654): 943–8, 1988. Mammographic screening and mortality from breast cancer: The Malmo mammographic screening trial. Andersson I, Aspegren K, Janzon L, Landberg T, Lindholm K, Linell F, Ljungberg O, Ranstam J, Sigfusson.

Br Med J 314: 925–928, 1997. Cohort study of association of risk of breast cancer with cyst type in women with gross cystic disease of the breast. Bruzzi P, Dogliotti L, Naldoni C, Bucchi L, Costantini M, Cicognani A, Torta M, Buzzi GF, Angeli A.

Breast J 1(2): 68–78, 1995. Ductal Carcinoma In Situ: Controversies in Diagnosis, Biology, and Treatment. Michael D, Lagios, MD.

Breast Cancer Res Treat 7: 45–46, 1986. Reduced recurrence-free survival after reduced doses of adjuvant chemotherapy in breast cancer: are groups selected after randomization comparable? Rutqvist LE, Wallgren A, Wennerholm AC.

Breast Cancer Res Treat 14: 140, 1989. Breast conservation treatment vs. modified modified radical mastectomy. Chaudry MA, Habib F, Tong D, Winter PJ, Fentiman IS, Hayward JL.

Breast Cancer Res Treat 21: 15–26, 1992. Endocrine therapy for advanced breast cancer: a review. Muss HB.

Breast Cancer Res Treat 29: 41–49, 1994. The epidermal growth factor receptor as a prognostic marker: results of 370 patients and review of 3009 patients. Fox SB, Smith K, Hollyer J, Greenall M, Hastrich D, Harris AL.

Breast Cancer Res Treat 29: 117–125, 1994. Epidermal growth factor receptor expression in breast cancer: association with response to endocrine therapy. Nicholson RI, McClelland RA, Gee JM, Manning DL, Cannon P, Robertson JF, Ellis IO, Blamey RW.

Breast Cancer Res Treat 37: 50, 1996. Incidence of axillary recurence after complete axillary dissection for breast cancer—15 years follow-up, Abstract. Singhal H, et al.

Breast Cancer Res Treat 41: 219(1), 1996. Does delaying breast irradiation in order to administer adjuvant chemotherapy increase the rate of ipsilateral breast tumor recurrence (BRT)? Results from two NSABP adjuvant studies in node positive breast cancer. Mamoumas EP, Fisher B, Bryant J, Wickerham DL, Brown A, Wolmark N.

Breast Cancer Res Treat; 45(3): 251–62, 1997. A phase III comparison of two toremifene doses to tamoxifen in postmenopausal women with advanced breast cancer Eastern European Study Group. Gershanovich M, Garin A, Baltina D, Kurvet A, Kangas L, Ellmen J.

Breast Cancer Res Treat 46: 8, 1997. Comparison of overall survival in two trials comparing letrozole 25 mg, Femara) with megestrol acetate or with aminoglutethimide in patients with advanced breast cancer. Smith IE, Chaudri HA, Lassus M, Hornberger U.

Breast Cancer Res Treat 46: 21, 1997. The natural history of breast cancer: What have we learned from screening? 16-year year follow-up of 2500 women, mortality and survival data, tumor progression, therapeutic implications. Tabar L.

Breast Cancer Res Treat 46: (Abs 16), 1997. The effect of increasing dose-intensity and cummulative dose of adjuvant cyclophosphamide in node (+) breast cancer: Results of NSABP-B25. Wolmark N, Fisher B, Anderson S.

Can Med Assoc J, 147: 1459–88, 1992. Canadian National Breast Cancer Screening Study. Miller AB, Baines CJ, To T, et al.

CA Cancer J Clin 42: 134–162, 1992. Standards for breast-conservation treatment, Winchester DP, Cox JD.

CA Cancer J Clin 45: 199–226, 1995. Current status of adjuvant systemic therapy for primary breast cancer: progress and controversy. Hortobagyi GN, Buzdar AU.

CA Cancer J Clin 45: 227–243, 1995. Primary chemotherapy in surgically resectable breast cancer. Bonadonna G, Valagussa P, Zucali R, Salvadori B.

CA Cancer J Clin 45: 263–278, 1995. The woman at increased risk for breast cancer: evaluation and management strategies. Bilimoria MM, Morrow M.

Cancer 36: 1603–1612, 1975. Intra-arterial infusion chemotherapy as preoperative treatment of locally advanced breast cancer. Koyama H, Wada T, Takahashi Y, Iwanaga T, Aoki Y.

Cancer 40: 1269–1275, 1977. Breast cancer incidence according to weight and height in two cities of the Netherlands and in Aichi prefecture, Japan. De Waard F, Cornelis JP, Aoki K, Yoshida M.

Cancer 41: 1170–1178, 1978. Patterns of relapse and survival following radical mastectomy Analysis of 716 consecutive patients. Valagussa P, Bonadonna G, Veronesi U.

Cancer 45: 2913–2916, 1980. Multicentricity of non-palpable breast cancer. Schwartz GF, Patchesfsky AS, Feig SA, Shaber GS, Schwartz AB.

Cancer 46: 647–653, 1980. A combined treatment program for the management of locally recurrent breast cancer following chest wall irradiation. Elkort RJ, Kelly W, Mozden PJ, Feldman MI.

Cancer 46: 2829–2834, 1980. Quantitative estrogen receptor analyses: the response to endocrine and cytotoxic chemotherapy in human breast cancer and the disease-free interval. Lippman ME, Allegra JC.

Cancer 47: 653–657, 1981. Phase II study: Intra-arterial BCNU therapy for metastatic brain tumors. Madajewicz S, West CR, Park HC, Ghoorah J, Avellanosa AM, Takita H, Karakousis C, Vincent R, Caracandas J, Jennings E.

Cancer 48: 1522–1527, 1981. One-day VATH (vinblastine, adriamycin, thiotepa and halotestin) therapy for advanced breast cancer refractory to chemotherapy. Hart RD, Perloff M, Halland JF.

Cancer 49: 217–220, 1982. A phase II study of combined 5-fluorouracil and mitomycin C in advanced breast cancer. Mattsson W, VanEyben F, Hallsten L, Bjelkengren G.

Cancer 49: 759–772, 1982. Diagnosis and treatment of leptomeningeal metastases from solid tumors: experience with 90 patients. Wasserstrom WR, Glass JP, Posner JB.

Cancer 50: 1309–1314, 1982. Duct carcinoma in situ Relationship of extent of noninvasive disease to the frequency of occult invasion, multicentricity, lymph node metastases, and short-term treatment failures. Lagios MD, Westdahl PR, Margolin FR, Rose MR.

Cancer 53: 712–723, 1984. Pathologic findings from the National Surgical Adjuvant Project for Breast Cancers, protocol no (4) X Discriminants for 10th year treatment failure. Fisher ER, Sass R, Fisher B.

Cancer 55: 658–665, 1985. Long-term survival of 458 young breast cancer patients. Rutqvist LE, Wallgren A.

Cancer 56: 225–229, 1985. Five-day continuous-infusion vinblastine in the treatment of breast cancer. Fraschini G, Yap H, Hortobagyi GN, Buzdar A, Blumenschein G.

Cancer 56: 979–990, 1985. Histologic multifocality of Tis, T1-2 breast carcinomas Implications for clinical trials of breast-conserving surgery. Holland R, Veling SH, Mravunac M, Hendriks JH.

Cancer 56: 1206–1208, 1985. Do regular ovulatory cycles increase breast cancer risk? Henderson BE, Ross RK, Judd HL, Krailo MD, Pike MC.

Cancer 59: 682–687, 1987. Distribution of axillary node metastases by level of invasion An analysis of 539 cases. Veronesi U, Rilke F, Luini A, Sacchini V, Galimberti V, Campa T, Dei Bei E, Greco M, Magni A, Merson M, et al.

Cancer 59: 1819–1824, 1987. Axillary lymph node dissection for intraductal breast carcinoma—is it indicated? Silverstein MJ, Rosser RJ, Gierson ED, Waisman JR, Gamagami P, Hoffman RS, Fingerhut AG, Lewinsky BS, Colburn W, Handel N.

Cancer 61: 1483–1491, 1988. Management of inflammatory carcinoma of the breast with combined modality therapy including intraarterial infusion chemotherapy as an induction therapy Long-term follow-up results of 28 patients. Noguchi S, Miyauchi K, Nishizawa Y, Koyama H, Terasawa T.

Cancer 62: 2226–2233, 1988. Metastatic pattern in recurrent breast cancer Special reference to intrathoracic recurrences. Kamby C, Vejborg I, Kristensen B, Olsen LO, Mouridsen HT.

Cancer 63: 37–45, 1989. Decreased cardiac toxicity of doxorubicin administered by continuous intravenous infusion in combination chemotherapy for metastatic breast carcinoma. Hortobagyi GN, Frye D, Buzdar AU, Ewer MS, Fraschini G, Hug V, Ames, Montague E, Carrasco CH, Mackay B, et al.

Cancer 63: 618–624, 1989. Mammographically detected duct carcinoma in situ Frequency of local recurrence following tylectomy and prognostic effect of nuclear grade on local recurrence. Lagios MD, Margolin FR, Westdahl PR, Rose MR.

Cancer 63: 1912–1917, 1989. Local recurrence after breast-conserving surgery and radiotherapy Frequency, time course, and prognosis. Kurtz JM, Amalric R, Brandone H, Ayme Y, Jacquemier J, Pietra JC, Hans D, Pollet JF, Bressac C, Spitalier JM.

Cancer 64: 1177–1182, 1989. The survival pattern in male breast cancer An analysis of 1429 patients from the Nordic countries. Adami HO, Hakulinen T, Ewertz M, Tretli S, Holmberg L, Karjalainen S.

Cancer 64: 1914–1921, 1989. Prognostic value of histologic grade nuclear components of Scarff-Bloom-Richardson (SBR) An improved score modification based on a multivariate analysis of 1262 invasive ductal breast carcinomas. Doussal Le, Tubiana-Hulin M, Friedman S, Hacene K, Spyratos F, Brunet M.

Cancer 66: 431–436, 1990. The Duke AFM Program: Intensive induction chemotherapy for metastatic breast cancer. Jones RB, Shpall EJ, Shogan J, et al.

Cancer 66: 645–650, 1990. Intraarterial induction chemotherapy in locally advanced stage III breast cancer. Stephens FO.

Cancer 67: 869–872, 1991. Prognosis of pregnancy-associated breast cancer. Petrek JA, Dukoff R, Rogatko A.

Cancer 67: 1685–1695, 1991. Meningeal carcinomatosis in breast cancer Prognostic factors and influence of treatment. Boogerd W, Hart AA, van der Sande JJ, Engelsman E.

Cancer 68: 2337–2344, 1991. Ten-year results of breast-conserving surgery and definitive irradiation for intraductal carcinoma, ductal carcinoma in situ) of the breast. Solin LJ, Recht A, Fourquet A, Kurtz K, Kuske R, McNeese M, McCormick B, Cross MA, Schultz DJ, Bornstein BA.

Cancer 69: 1885–1887, 1992. American Cancer Society Guidelines on Screening for Breast Cancer. Dodd GD.

Cancer 70: 2468–2474, 1992. Subclinical ductal carcinoma in situ of the breast Treatment by local excision and surveillance alone. Schwartz GF, Finkel GC, Garcia JC, Patchefsky AS.

Cancer 71: 1254–1257, 1993. Phase II trial of carboplatin and etoposide in metastatic breast Cancer. Crown J, Hakes T, Reichman B, Lebwohl D, Gilewski T, Surbone A, Currie V, Yao TJ, Hudis C, Seidman A, et al.

Cancer 71: 1258–1265, 1993. Breast cancer risk associated with proliferative breast disease and atypical hyperplasia. Dupont WD, Parl FF, Hartmann WH, Brinton LA, Winfield AC, Worrell JA, Schuyler PA, Plummer WD.

Cancer 71: 1797–1800, 1993. Typhlitis resulting from treatment with taxol and doxorubicin in patients with metastatic breast cancer. Pestalozzi BC, Sotos GA, Choyke PL, Fisherman JS, Cowan KH, O'Shaughnessy JA.

Cancer 71: 3054–3057, 1993. Lung Cancer after radiation therapy for breast cancer. Neugut AI, Robinson E, Lee WC, Murray T, Karwoski K, Kutcher GJ.

Cancer 72: 1457–1460, 1993. Breast cancer detection in an institution Is mammography detrimental? Kopans DB.

Cancer 73: 1836–1841, 1994. Breast cancer diagnosis by lactate dehydrogenase isozymes in nipple discharge. Kawamoto M, Kawamoto G.

Cancer 74(1 Suppl): 416–23, 1994. Multidisciplinary management of advanced primary and metastatic breast cancer. Hortobagyi GN.

Cancer 74: 1360–1366, 1994. A radiologic syndrome after high dose chemotherapy and autologous bone marrow transplantation, with clinical and pathologic features of systemic candidiasis. Mudad R, Vredenburgh J, Paulson EK, Ross M, Meisenberg B, Hussein A, Peters WP.

Cancer 74: 1746–1751, 1994. The relationship between microscopic margins of resection and the risk of local recurrence in patients with breast cancer treated with breast-conserving surgery and radiation therapy. Schnitt SJ, Abner A, Gelman R, Connolly JL, Recht A, Duda RB, Eberlein TJ, Mayzel K, Silver B, Harris JR.

Cancer 75: 1310–1319, 1995. Pathologic findings from the National Surgical Adjuvant Breast Project, NSABP) Protocol B-17 Intraductal carcinoma, ductal carcinoma in situ. The National Surgical Adjuvant Breast and Bowel Project Collaborating Investigators. Fisher ER, Costantino J, Fisher B, Palekar AS, Redmond C, Mamounas E.

Cancer 76(2): 275–283, 1995. Better breast cancer survival for postmenopausal women who are less overweight and eat less fat. The Iowa Women's Health Study. Zhang S, Folsom AR, Sellers TA, Kushi LH, Potter JD.

Cancer 77(11): 2267–2274, 1996. A prognostic index for ductal carcinoma in situ of the breast. Silverstein MJ, Lagios MD, Craig PH, Waisman JR, Lewinsky BS, Colburn WJ, Poller DN.

Cancer 77(12): 2496–2502, 1996. Radiation-associated angiosarcoma: diagnostic and thera-peutic implications-two case reports and a review of the literature. Cafiero F, Gipponi M, Peressini A, Queirolo P, Bertoglio S, Comandini D, Percivale P, Sertoli MR, Badellino F.

Cancer 78(5): 1024–1034, 1996. Lobular neoplasia Long term risk of breast cancer and relation to other factors. Bodian CA, Perzin KH, Lattes R.

Cancer 79: 1362–1369, 1997. Breast conserving therapy for stage I–II synchronous bilateral breast carcinoma. Gollamudi SV, Gelman RS, Peiro G, Schneider LH, Schnitt SJ, Recht A, Silver BJ, Harris JR, Connolly JL.

Cancer 80(11): 2091–2099, 1997. The Gothenburg breast screening trial: first results on mortality, incidence, and mode of detection for women ages 39–49 years at randomization. Bjurstam N, Bjorneld L, Duffy SW, Smith TC, Cahlin E, Eriksson O, Hafstrom LO, Lingaas H, Mattsson J, Persson S, Rudenstam CM, Save-Soderbergh J.

Cancer 83(6) Sep 15: 1142–1152, 1998. Anastrozole versus megestrol acetate in the treatment of postmenopausal women with advanced breast carcinoma: results of a survival update based on a combined analysis of data from two mature phase III trials. Arimidex Study Group. Buzdar AU, Jonat W, Howell A, Jones SE, Blomqvist CP, Vogel CL, Eiermann W, Wolter JM, Steinberg M, Webster A, Lee D.

Cancer 82(12): 2382–2390, 15 June 1998. Mammary ductal carcinoma in situ with microinvasion. Silver SA, Tavassoli FA.

Cancer Causes Control 5: 73–82, 1994. Alcoholic beverage consumption in relation to risk of breast cancer. Longnecker MP.

Cancer Causes Control 7: 539–543, 1996. Laterality of breast cancer in the US. Weiss HA, Devesa SS, Brinton LA.

Cancer Invest 6(3): 245–254, 1988. Menstrual factors and risk of breast cancer. Brinton LA, et al.

Cancer Invest 8: 327–334, 1990. Combination therapy with platinum and etoposide of brain metastases from breast carcinoma. Cocconi G, Lottici R, Bisagni G, Bacchi M, Tonato M, Passalacqua R, Boni C, Belsanti V, Bassi P.

Cancer Invest 9: 249–255, 1991. Combination chemotherapy with cyclophosphamide, fluorouracil, and either epirubicin or mitoxantrone: a comparative randomized multicenter study in metastatic breast carcinoma. Periti P, Pannuti F, Della Cuna GR, Mazzei T, Mini E, Martoni A, Preti P, Ercolino L, Pavesi L, Ribecco A.

Cancer Invest 12: 17–18, 1994. Navelbine: A promising new drug with favorable toxicity profile for breast cancer and non-small cell lung cancer (NSCLC). Vogel CL, Bertsch LA, Hohneker JA.

Cancer Invest 12: 30–33, 1994. Taxol. Helson L, Hortobagyi GN, Chang AY.

Cancer Invest 12: 35–36, 1994. Taxotere in breast cancer. Trudeau M.

Cancer Invest 12: 38, 1994. Pharmacogenetics of amonafide: An active drug in breast cancer? Ratain MJ.

Cancer Invest 12: 63–64, 1994. Liposomal doxorubicin in experimental and clinical breast and lung cancer. Batist G.

Cancer Invest 13: 381–404, 1995. Taxanes, a new class of antitumor agents. Huizing MT, Misser VH, Pieters RC.

Cancer Invest 13, (suppl 1): 29–30, 1995. Phase II study of TLC D-99, Liposomal doxorubicin), 5-FU, cyclophosphamide in patients with metastatic breat cancer. Valero V, Buzdar A, Walters R, Willey J, et al.

Cancer Invest 15: 475–90, 1997. Vinorelbine (Navelbine): a third generation vinca alkaloid (review).

Cancer J Sci Am 2(3): 158, May 1996. Mammographically Detected, Clinically Occult Ductal Carcinoma In Situ Treated With Breast-Conserving Surgery and Definitive Breast Irradiation. Solin LJ, McCormick B, Recht A, Haffty BG, Taylor ME, Kuske RR, Bornstein BA, McNeese M, Schultz DJ, Fowble BL, Barrett W, Yeh IT, Kurtz JM, Amalric R, Fourquet A.

Cancer Res 2: 468–475, 1942. The genesis and growth of tumors. Tannenbaum A.

Cancer Res 42: 4788–4791, 1982. Tamoxifen and oophorectomy in the treatment of recurrent breast cancer: a Southwest Oncology Group Study. Hoogstraten B, Fletcher WS, Gad-el-Mawla N, Maloney T, Altman SJ, Vaughn CB, Foulkes MA.

Cancer Res 46(6): 3152–3156, June 1986. Role and mechanism of action of tamoxifen in premenopausal women with metastatic breast carcinoma. Sawka CA, Pritchard KI, Paterson AH, Sutherland DJ, Thomson DB, Shelley WE, Myers RE, Mobbs BG, Malkin A, Meakin JW.

Cancer Res 51: 556–567, 1991. Correlation between c-erbB-2 amplification and risk of recurrent disease in node-negative breast cancer. Paterson MC, Dietrich KD, Danyluk J, Paterson AH, Lees AW, Jamil N, Hanson J, Jenkins H, Krause BE, McBlain WA, et al.

Cancer Res 52: 2127–2137, 1992. Evolving concepts in the systemic adjuvant treatment of breast cancer. Bonadonna G.

Cancer Res 54: 5875–5881, 1994. Clinical and endocrine effects of the oral aromatase inhibitor vorozole in postmenopausal patients with advanced breast cancer. Johnston SR, Smith IE, Doody D, Jacobs S, Robertshaw H, Dowsett M.

Cancer Res Ther Control 4(1): 43–7, 1994. Advances in the detection of marrow micrometastases in breast cancer (Meeting abstract). Abou Ghalia A, Silva O, Vredenburgh JJ, Bast RC, Jr.

Cancer Treat Rep 60(6): 665–698, 1976. Nitrosoureas: a review of experimental antitumor activity. Schabel FM, Jr.

Cancer Treat Rep 64: 787–796, 1980. Tamoxifen therapy in premenopausal patients with metastatic breast cancer. Pritchard KI, Thomson DB, Myers RE, Sutherland DJ, Mobbs BG, Meakin JW.

Cancer Treat Rep 67(4): 343–350, 1983. Cardiac evaluation of mitoxantrone. Unverferth DV, Unverferth BJ, Balcerzak SP, Bashore TA, Neidhart JA.

Cancer Treat Rep 71(1): 15–29, January 1987. Overview of randomized trials of postoperative adjuvant radiotherapy in breast cancer Cuzick J, Stewart H, Peto R, Baum M, Fisher B, Host H, Lythgoe JP, Ribeiro G, Scheurlen H, Wallgren A.

Cancer Treat Res 61: 59–68, 1992. The role of the retinoblastoma gene in breast cancer development. Fung YK, T'Ang A.

Cancer Treat Rev 18: 261–276, 1991. Eye metastasis from carcinoma of the breast: diagnosis, radiation treatment and results. Ratanatharathorn V, Powers WE, Grimm J, Steverson N, Han I, Ahmad K, Lattin PB.

Cancer Treat Rev 19: 105–112, 1993. Menstrual effects on surgical treatment for breast cancer. Davidson NE, Abeloff MD.

Cell 79: 315–328, 1994. Angiostatin: a novel angiogenesis inhibitor that mediates the suppression of metastases by a Lewis lung carcinoma. O'Reilly, MS, Holmgren L, Shing Y, Chen C, Rosenthal RA, Moses M, Lane WS, Cao Y, Sage EH, Folkman J.

Chest 102: 1113–1117, 1992. Pulmonary lymphangitic metastasis from breast cancer Lymphocytic alveolitis is associated with favorable prognosis. Lower E, Baughman RP.

Clin Genet 29: 222–233, 1986. The Cowden syndrome: a clinical and genetic study in 21 patients. Starink PM, van der Veen JP, Arwert F, deWaal LP, deLange GG, Gille JJ, et al.

Contemporary Oncology 4: 23–31, Janaury 1994. Hereditary Breast Cancer.

Contemporary Surgery 49(1): 37–50, 1996. Symposium: Management of ductal carcinoma in situ and lobular carcinoma in situ. Moderator, Kirby Bland, MD, Panelists were: Kinne D, Suzanne Klimberg V, Singletary SE.

Contemporary Surgery 49(2): 71–75, 1996. A statewide review of male breast carcinoma Male Breast Cancer. Lipshy K, Denning D, Wheeler W.

Contraception 40: 1–38, 1989. Cancer of the breast and reproductive tract in relation to use of oral contraceptives. Schlesselman JJ.

Curr Opin Oncol 9(6): 527–531, 1997. Radiation therapy and breast cancer, Gage I, Harris J.

Curr Opin Oncol 9(6): 532–539, November 1997. Systemic therapy for breast cancer. Kennedy MJ.

Current Opinion in Oncology 9(6): 584–589, 1997. Clinical trails of antiangiogenic agents, Twardowski P, Gradishar W.

Cytometry 14: 482–485, 1993. Consensus review of the clinical utility of DNA cytometry in carcinoma of the breastReport of the DNA Cytometry Consensus Conference. Hedley DW, Clark GM, Cornelisse CJ, Killander D, Kute T, Merkel D.

Diagn Imaging Clin Med 54(3–4): 178–85, 1985. The role of specimen X-ray in the diagnosis of breast cancer. Holland R.

Drugs 45: 20–30, 1993. Epirubicin Clinical pharmacology and dose-effect relationship. Robert J.

Epidemiology 6: 137–141, 1995. A meta-analysis of body mass index and risk of premenopausal breast cancer. Ursin G, Longnecker MP, Haile RW, Greenland S.

Epidemiology 8: 181–187, 1997. Prenatal and perinatal risk factors for breast cancer in young women, Weiss HA, Potischman NA, Brinton, LA, Brogan D, Coates RJ, Gammon MD, Malone KE, Schoenberg JB.

Epidemiol Rev, (Engl Transl Przegl Epidemiol), 1:74–109, 1979. A review of the epidemiology of human breast cancer. Kelsey JL.

Epidemiol Rev 15(1): 17–35, 1993. Estrogens, progestogens, normal breast cell proliferation, and breast cancer risk. Pike MC, Spicer DV, Dahmoush L, Press MF.

Epidemiol Rev 15: 157–62, 1993. Radiation and other environmental exposures and breast cancer. John EM, Kelsey JL.

Eur J Cancer 26(6): 668–670, 1990. Breast conservation is the treatment of choice in small breast cancer: long-term results of a randomized trial. Veronesi U, Banfi A, Salvadori B, Luini A, Saccozzi R, Zucali R, Marubini E, Del Vecchio M, Boracchi P, Marchini S, et al.

Eur J Cancer 26(6): 671–673, 1990. Quadrantectomy versus lumpectomy for small size breast cancer. Veronesi U, Volterrani F, Luini A, Saccozzi R, Del Vecchio M, Zucali R, Galimberti V, Rasponi A, Di Re E, Squicciarini P, et al.

Eur J Cancer 27: 220–221, 1991. Interferon plus dacarbazine in advanced malignant melanoma: a phase I–II study. Gundersen S, Flokkmann A.

Eur J Cancer 28(2–3): 630–634, 1992. Duct carcinoma in situ: 227 cases without microinvasion. Silverstein MJ, Cohlan BF, Gierson ED, Furmanski M, Gamagami P, Colburn WJ, Lewinsky BS, Waisman JR.

Eur J Cancer 28A: 810–814, 1992. Goserelin depot in the treatment of premenopausal advanced breast cancer. Blamey RW, Jonat W, Kaufmann M, Bianco AR, Namer M.

Eur J Cancer 28A: 1941–1945, 1992. 4-hydroxyandrostenedione: a new treatment for postmenopausal patients with breast cancer. Coombes RC, Hughes SW, Dowsett M.

Eur J Cancer 29a(8): 1093–1096, 1993. Central small size breast cancer: How to overcome the problem of nipple and areolar involvement. Galimberti V, Zurrida S, Zanini V, Callegari M, Veronesi P, Catania S, Luini A, Greco M, Grisotti A.

Eur J Cancer; 29A(13): 1824–31 1993. Sarcomatoid tumours of the breast in Denmark from 1977 to 1987: A clinicopathological and immunohistochemical study of 100 cases. Christensen L, Schidt T, Blichert-Toft M.

Eur J Cancer 30A(5): 645–652, 1994. Neoadjuvant versus adjuvant chemotherapy in premenopausal patients with tumours considered too large for breast conserving surgery: preliminary results of a randomised trial: S6. Scholl SM, Fourquet A, Asselain B, Pierga JY, Vilcoq JR, Durand JC, Dorval T, Palangie T, Jouve M, Beuzeboc P, et al.

Eur J Cancer; 31A Suppl 4: S11–3, 1995. An overview of phase II studies of docetaxel in patients with metastatic breast cancer, Eisenhauer EA, Trudeau M.

Eur J Cancer 31A(10): 1574–1579, September 1995. Breast conservation is a safe method in patients with small cancer of the breast Long-term results of three randomised trials on 1973 patients. Istituto Nazionale per lo Studio e la Cura dei Tumori, Milano, Italy. Veronesi U, Salvadori B, Luini A, Greco M, Saccozzi R, del Vecchio M, Mariani L, Zurrida S, Rilke F.

Eur J Cancer 32A: 404–412, 1996. A randomised trial comparing two doses of the new selective aromatase inhibitor anastrozole, (Arimidex) with megestrol acetate in postmenopausal patients with advanced breast cancer. Jonat W, Howell A, Blomqvist C, Eiermann W, Winblad G, Tyrrell C, Mauriac L, Roche H, Lundgren S, Hellmund R, Azab M.

Eur J Cancer 32A: 2528–2533, 1996. Experimental and clinical studies on the use of matrix metalloproteinase inhibitors in the for the treatment of cancer. Talbot DC, Brown PD.

Eur J Cancer 33(2): 193–199, 1997. Arm morbidity after sector resection and axillary dissection with or without postoperative radiotherapy in breast cancer stage I Results from a randomised trial Uppsala-Orebro Breast Cancer Study Group. Liljegren G, Holmberg L.

Eur J Cancer Prev 5(6): 476–82, 1996. Hormonal events during female puberty in relation to breast cancer risk. Apter D.

Eur J Surg Oncol 14: 311–316, 1988. Polyadenylic-polyuridylic acid as adjuvant in the treatment of operable breast cancer: recent results. Lacour J, Lacour F, Ducot B, Spira A, Michelson M, Petit JY, Sarrazin D, Contesso G.

Eur J Surg Oncol 15: 25–31, 1989. Histological grading of breast cancer; significance of grade on recurrence and mortality. Hopton DS, Thorogood J, Clayden AD, MacKinnon D.

Eur J Surg Oncol 20: 641–643, 1994. Surgical pitfalls after preoperative chemotherapy in large size breast cancer. Zurrida S, Greco M, Veronesi U.

Fertil Steril 61(1): 178–180, 1994. Comparative study: Replens versus local estrogen in menopausal women. Nachtigall LE.

Fertil Steril 68(6): 981–986, 1997. Does dong quai have estrogenic effects in postmenopausal women? A double-blind, placebo-controlled trial. Hirata JD, Swiersz LM, Zell B, Small R, Ettinger B.

Gene 159: 19–27, 1995. The c-erbB-2 proto-oncogene as a prognostic and predictive marker in breast cancer: a paradigm for the development of other macromolecular markers—a review. Ravdin PM, Chamness GC.

Gynecol Oncol 55: 164–168, 1994. Tamoxifen use in breast cancer patients who subsequently develop corpus cancer is not associated with a higher incidence of adverse histologic features. Barakat RR, Wong G, Curtin JP, Vlamis V, Hoskins WJ.

Hum Mol Genet 2: 1799–1802, 1993. Androgen receptor gene mutation in male breast cancer. Lobaccaro JM, Lumbroso S, Belon C, Galtier-Dereure F, Bringer J, Lesimple T, et al.

Int J Cancer; 70(2): 164–8, 1997. Breast-cancer mortality in a non-randomized trial on mammographic screening in women over age 65. Van Dijck JA, Verbeek AL, Beex LV, Hendriks JH, Holland R, Mravunac M, Straatman H, Werre JM.

Int J Radiat Oncol Biol Phys 12: 727–732, 1986. Postoperative radiotherapy in breast cancer: long-term results from the Oslo study. Host H, Brennhovd IO, Loeb M.

Int J Radiat Oncol Biol Phys 15: 627–631, 1988. Radiotherapy for the prevention of local- regional recurrence in high risk patients post mastectomy receiving adjuvant chemotherapy. Fowble B, Glick J, Goodman R.

Int J Radiat Oncol Biol Phys 15: 711–716, 1988. Hyperthermia in combination with definitive radiation therapy: results of a Phase I/II RTOG Study. Scott R, Gillespie B, Perez CA, Hornback NB, Johnson R, Emami B, Bauer M, Pakuris E.

Int J Radiat Oncol Biol Phys 17: 719–725, 1989. Prognostic factors of breast recurrence in the conservative management of early breast cancer: a 25-year follow-up. Fourquet A, Campana F, Zafrani B, Mosseri V, Vielh P, Durand JC, Vilcoq JR.

Int J Radiat Oncol Biol Phys 23: 915–923, 1992. Long-term radiation complications following conservative surgery (CS) and radiation therapy, RT) in patients with early stage breast cancer. Pierce SM, Recht A, Lingos TI, Abner A, Vicini F, Silver B, Herzog A, Harris JR.

Int J Radiat Oncol Biol Phys 25: 79–85, 1993. Local hyperthermia, radiation therapy, and chemotherapy in patients with local-regional recurrence of breast carcinoma. Bornstein BA, Zouranjian PS, Hansen JL, Fraser SM, Gelwan LA, Teicher BA, Svensson GK.

Int J Radiat Oncol Biol Phys 30;26(1): 135–139, April 1993.
Angiosarcoma of the breast following lumpectomy, axillary lymph node
dissection, and radiotherapy for primary breast cancer: three case reports
and a review of the literature. Wijnmaalen A, van Ooijen B, van Geel
BN, Henzen-Logmans SC, Treurniet-Donker AD.

Int J Radiat Oncol Biol Phys 35(4): 649–659, 1 July 1996. Timing of
radiotherapy and chemotherapy following breast-conserving surgery for
patients with node-positive breast cancer. International Breast Cancer
Study Group. Wallgren A, Bernier J, Gelber RD, Goldhirsch A,
Roncadin M, Joseph D, Castiglione-Gertsch M.

Int J Radiat Oncol Biol Phys 35(4): 731–744, 1 July 1996.
Radiotherapy with or without hyperthermia in the treatment of
superficial localized breast cancer: results from five randomized
controlled trials. International Collaborative Hyperthermia Group.
Vernon CC, Hand JW, Field SB, Machin D, Whaley JB, van der
Zee J, van Putten WL, van Rhoon GC, van Dijk JD, Gonzalez
Gonzalez D, Liu FF, Goodman P, Sherar M.

Int J Radiat Oncol Biol Phys 35(5): 1117–1121, 15 July 1996. Efficacy
of adjuvant hyperthermia in the treatment of superficial recurrent breast
cancer: confirmation and future directions. Kapp DS.

Int J Radiat Oncol Biol Phys 38(3): 541–550, 1 June 1997.
Long-term follow-up of axillary node-positive breast cancer patients
receiving adjuvant systemic therapy alone: patterns of recurrence.
Fisher BJ, Perera FE, Cooke AL, Opeitum A, Venkatesan V, Dar AR,
Stitt L.

Int J Radiat Oncol Biol Phys 39(5):1069–1076, 1 December 1997. The
role of regional nodal irradiation in the management of patients with
early-stage breast cancer treated with breast-conserving therapy Vicini
FA, Horwitz EM, Lacerna MD, Brown DM, White J, Dmuchowski CF,
Kini VR, Martinez A.

J Am Acad Dermatol 11(6): 1127–41, 1984. Cowden's disease: analysis
of fourteen new cases. Starink TM.

J Am Coll Surg 183(6): 575–582, December 1996. Therapeutic options and results for the management of minimally invasive carcinoma of the breast: influence of axillary dissection for treatment of T1a and T1b lesions. White RE, Vezeridis MP, Konstadoulakis M, Cole BF, Wanebo HJ, Bland KI.

J Am Coll Surg 184: 493–498, 1997. Axillary lymph node dissection: Is it required in T1a breast cancer? Chontos AJ, Maher DP, Ratzer ER, Fenoglio ME.

J Am Med Assoc 260(5): 652–6, 1988. A Meta-analysis of alcohol consumption in relation to risk of breast cancer. Longnecker MP, Berlin JA, Orza MJ, Chalmers TC.

J Am Med Assoc 276(22): 1818–1822, 1996. Lymphatic mapping and sentinel node biopsy in the patient with breast cancer. Albertini JJ, Lyman GH, Cox C, Yeatman T, Balducci L, Ku N, Shivers S, Berman C, Wells K, Rapaport D, Shons A, Horton J, Greenberg H, Nicosia S, Clark R, Cantor A, Reintgen DS.

J Am Med Assoc 279(7): 535–540, 1998. Alcohol and breast cancer in women: a pooled analysis of cohort studies. Smith-Warner SA, et al.

J Clin Oncol 1: 2–10, 1983. Adjuvant CMF in breast cancer: comparative 5-year results of 12 versus six cycles. Tancini G, Bonadonna G, Valagussa P, Marchini S, Veronesi U.

J Clin Oncol 3: 1640–1658, 1985. Leukemia in breast cancer patients following adjuvant chemotherapy or postoperative radiation: the NSABP experience. Fisher B, Rockette H, Fisher ER, Wickerham DL, Redmond C, Brown A.

J Clin Oncol 4: 178–185, 1986. Randomized trial of bilateral oophorectomy versus tamoxifen in premenopausal women with metastatic breast cancer. Ingle JN, Krook JE, Green SJ, Kubista TP, Everson LK, Ahmann DL, Chang MN, Bisel HF, Windschitl HE, Twito DI, et al.

J Clin Oncol 4: 459–471, 1986. Adjuvant chemotherapy with and without tamoxifen in the treatment of primary breast cancer: 5-year results from the National Surgical Adjuvant Breast and Bowel Project Trial. Fisher , Redmond C, Brown A, Fisher ER, Wolmark N, Bowman D, Plotkin D, Wolter J, Bornstein R, Legault-Poisson S, et al.

J Clin Oncol 4: 958–964, 1986. Randomized trial of tamoxifen alone or combined with aminoglutethimide and hydrocortisone in women with metastatic breast cancer. Ingle JN, Green SJ, Ahmann DL, Long HJ, Edmonson JH, Rubin J, Chang MN, Creagan ET.

J Clin Oncol 4: 1326–1330, 1986. A randomized comparison of tamoxifen with surgical oophorectomy in premenopausal patients with advanced breast cancer. Buchanan RB, Blamey RW, Durrant KR, Howell A, Paterson AG, Preece PE, Smith DC, Williams CJ, Wilson RG.

J Clin Oncol 4: 1542–1550, 1986. Comparison of circulating CA15-3 and carcinoembryonic antigen levels in patients with breast cance. Hayes DF, Zurawski VR, Kufe DW.

J Clin Oncol 5: 55–61, 1987. Survival from first recurrence: relative importance of prognostic factors in 1,015 breast cancer patients. Clark GM, Sledge GW, Osborne CK, McGuire WL.

J Clin Oncol 6: 1368–1376, 1988. High-dose combination alkylating agents with bone marrow support as initial treatment for metastatic breast cancer. Peters WP, Shpall EJ, Jones RB, Olsen GA, Bast RC, Gockerman JP, Moore JO.

J Clin Oncol 7: 560–571, 1989. Randomized clinical trial comparing mitoxantrone with doxorubicin in previously treated patients with metastatic breast cancer. Henderson IC, Allegra JC, Woodcock T, Wolff S, Bryan S, Cartwright K, Dukart G, Henry D.

J Clin Oncol 7: 572–582, 1989. Doxorubicin-containing regimens for the treatment of stage II breast cancer: The National Surgical Adjuvant Breast and Bowel Project experience. Fisher B, Redmond C, Wickerham DL, Bowman D, Schipper H, Wolmark N, Sass R, Fisher ER, Jochimsen P, Legault-Poisson S, et al.

J Clin Oncol 7: 879–889, 1989. Six-year results of the Eastern Cooperative Oncology Group trial of observation versus CMFP versus CMFPT in postmenopausal patients with node-positive breast cancer. Taylor SG, Knuiman MW, Sleeper LA, Olson JE, Tormey DC, Gilchrist KW, Falkson G, Rosenthal SN, Carbone PP, Cummings FJ.

J Clin Oncol 7: 1113–1119, 1989. Goserelin, a depot gonadotrophin-releasing hormone agonist in the treatment of premenopausal patients with metastatic breast cancer German Zoladex Trial Group. Kaufmann M, Jonat W, Kleeberg U, Eiermann W, Janicke F, Hilfrich J, Kreienberg R, Albrecht M, Weitzel HK, Schmid H, et al.

J Clin Oncol 8: 1483–1496, 1990. Two months of doxorubicin-cyclophosphamide with and without interval reinduction therapy compared with 6 months of cyclophosphamide, methotrexate, and fluorouracil in positive-node breast cancer patients with tamoxifen-nonresponsive tumors: results from the National Surgical Adjuvant Breast and Bowel Project B-15. Fisher B, Brown AM, Dimitrov NV, Poisson R, Redmond C, Margolese RG, Bowman D, Wolmark N, Wickerham DL, Kardinal CG, et al.

J Clin Oncol 8: 1005–1018, 1990. Postoperative chemotherapy and tamoxifen compared with tamoxifen alone in the treatment of positive-node breast cancer patients aged 50 years and older with tumors responsive to tamoxifen: results from the National Surgical Adjuvant Breast and Bowel Project B-16. Fisher B, Redmond C, Legault-Poisson S, Dimitrov NV, Brown AM, Wickerham DL, Wolmark N, Margolese, Bowman D, Glass AG, et al.

J Clin Oncol 8(7): 1207–1216, July 1990. Treatment of estrogen receptor-negative or hormonally refractory breast cancer with double high-dose chemotherapy intensification and bone marrow support. Dunphy FR, Spitzer G, Buzdar AU, Hortobagyi GN, Horwitz LJ, Yau JC, Spinolo JA, Jagannath S, Holmes F, Wallerstein RO, et al.

J Clin Oncol 8: 1217–1225, 1990. A randomized trial comparing 12 weeks versus 36 weeks of adjuvant chemotherapy in stage II breast cancer. Levine MN, Gent M, Hryniuk WM, Bramwell V, Abu-Zahra H, DePauw S, Arnold A, Findlay B, Levin L, Skillings J, et al.

J Clin Oncol 8: 1310–1320, 1990. Chemotherapy vs. tamoxifen vs. chemotherapy plus tamoxifen in node positive, estrogen receptor-positive breast cancer patients: results of a multicentric Italian study Breast Cancer Adjuvant Chemo–Hormone Therapy Cooperative Group. Boccardo F, Rubagotti A, Bruzzi P, Cappellini M, Isola G, Nenci I, Piffanelli A, Scanni A, Sismondi P, Santi L, et al.

J Clin Oncol 9: 664–669, 1991. Cisplatin and etoposide as first-line chemotherapy for metastatic breast carcinoma: a prospective randomized trial of the Italian Oncology Group for Clinical Research. Cocconi G, Bisagni G, Bacchi M, Boni C, Bartolucci R, Ceci G, Colozza MA, Lisi De, Lottici R, Mosconi AM, et al.

J Clin Oncol 9: 1283–1297, 1991. Tamoxifen in premenopausal patients with metastatic breast cancer: a review. Sunderland MC, Osborne CK.

J Clin Oncol 9: 1731–1735, 1991. Mitoxantrone, fluorouracil, and high-dose leucovorin: an effective, well-tolerated regimen for metastatic breast cancer. Hainsworth JD, Andrews MB, Johnson DH, Greco FA.

J Clin Oncol 9: 1749–1756, 1991. Prediction of early relapse in patients with operable breast cancer by detection of occult bone marrow micrometastases. Cote RJ, Rosen PP, Lesser ML, Old LJ, Osborne MP.

J Clin Oncol 9: 2016–2020, 1991. Mesna vs. hyperhydration for the prevention of cyclophosphamide-induced hemorrhagic cystitis in bone marrow transplantation. Shepherd JD, Pringle LE, Barnett MJ, Klingemann HG, Reece DE, Phillips GL.

J Clin Oncol 9: 2134–2140, 1991. Adjuvant chemotherapy with doxorubicin plus cyclophosphamide, methotrexate, and fluorouracil in the treatment of resectable breast cancer with more than three positive axillary nodes. Buzzoni R, Bonadonna G, Valagussa P, Zambetti M.

J Clin Oncol 9: 2153–2161, 1991. Factors predicting for response, time to treatment failure, and survival in women with metastatic breast cancer treated with DAVTH: a prospective Eastern Cooperative Oncology Group study. Falkson G, Gelman R, Falkson CI, Glick J, Harris J.

J Clin Oncol 10: 117–127, 1992. ICRF-187 permits longer treatment with doxorubicin in women with breast cancer. Speyer JL, Green MD, Zeleniuch-Jacquotte A, Wernz JC, Rey M, Sanger J, Kramer E, Ferrans V, Hochster H, Meyers M, et al.

J Clin Oncol 10: 976–983, 1992. Mastectomy versus breast-conserving therapy in the treatment of stage I and II carcinoma of the breast: a randomized trial at the National Cancer Institute. Lichter AS, Lippman ME, Danforth DN, d'Angelo T, Steinberg SM, deMoss E, MacDonald HD, Reichert CM, Merino M, Swain SM, et al.

J Clin Oncol 10: 984–989, 1992. Low-dose aminoglutethimide with and without hydrocortisone replacement as a first-line endocrine treatment in advanced breast cancer: a prospective randomized trial of the Italian Oncology Group for Clinical Research. Cocconi G, Bisagni G, Ceci G, Bacchi M, Boni C, Brugia M, Carpi A, Di Costanzo F, Franciosi V, Gori S, et al.

J Clin Oncol 10: 1014–1024, 1992. Inflammatory breast cancer: a review. Jaiyesimi IA, Buzdar AU, Hortobagyi G.

J Clin Oncol 10: 1049–1056, 1992. Prognostic importance of c-erbB-2 expression in breast cancer International, Ludwig) Breast Cancer Study Group. Gusterson BA, Gelber RD, Goldhirsch A, Price KN, Save-Soderborgh J, Anbazhagan R, Styles J, Rudenstam CM, Golouh R, Reed R, et al.

J Clin Oncol 10: 1674–1681, 1992. Breast cancer in patients irradiated for Hodgkin's disease: a clinical and pathologic analysis of 45 events in 37 patients. Yahalom J, Petrek JA, Biddinger PW, Kessler S, Dershaw D, McCormick B, Osborne MP, Kinne DA, Rosen PP.

J Clin Oncol 10(11): 1743–1747, 1992. High-dose consolidation therapy with autologous stem-cell rescue in stage IV breast cancer: follow-up report. Williams SF, Gilewski T, Mick R, Bitran JD.

J Clin Oncol 10(11): 1795–1801, 1992. Cardiotoxicity of high-dose continuous infusion fluorouracil: a prospective clinical study. de Forni M, Malet-Martino MC, Jaillais P, Shubinski RE, Bachaud JM, Lemaire L, Canal P, Chevreau C, Carrie D, Soulie P, et al.

J Clin Oncol 11: 561–569, 1993. Randomized prospective comparison of intraventricular methotrexate and thiotepa in patients with previously untreated neoplastic meningitis Eastern Cooperative Oncology Group. Grossman SA, Finkelstein DM, Ruckdeschel JC, Trump DL, Moynihan T, Ettinger DS.

J Clin Oncol 11: 1132–1143, 1993. High-dose chemotherapy and autologous bone marrow support as consolidation after standard-dose adjuvant therapy for high-risk primary breast cancer. Peters WP, Ross M, Vredenburgh JJ, Meisenberg B, Marks LB, Winer E, Kurtzberg J, Bast RC, Jones R, Shpall E, et al.

J Clin Oncol 11: 1529–1535, 1993. Phase II study of goserelin for patients with postmenopausal metastatic breast cancer. Saphner T, Troxel AM, Tormey DC, Neuberg D, Robert NJ, Pandya KJ, Edmonson JH, Rosenbluth RJ, Abeloff MD.

J Clin Oncol 11: 2090–2100, 1993. Factors influencing prognosis in node-negative breast carcinoma: analysis of 767 T1N0M0/T2N0M0 patients with long-term follow-up. Rosen PP, Groshen S, Kinne DW, Norton L.

J Clin Oncol 12: 447–453, 1994. Cause-specific mortality in long-term survivors of breast cancer who participated in trials of radiotherapy. Cuzick J, Stewart H, Rutqvist L, Houghton J, Edwards R, Redmond C, Peto R, Baum M, Fisher B, Host H, et al.

J Clin Oncol 12: 454–466, 1994. Tumor microvessel density, p53 expression, tumor size, and peritumoral lymphatic vessel invasion are relevant prognostic markers in node-negative breast carcinoma. Gasparini G, Weidner N, Bevilacqua P, Maluta S, Dalla Palma P, Caffo O, Barbareschi M, Boracchi P, Marubini E, Pozza F.

J Clin Oncol 12: 467–474, 1994. Cathepsin D by western blotting and immuno-histochemistry: failure to confirm correlations with prognosis in node-negative breast cancer. Ravdin PM, Tandon AK, Allred DC, Clark GM, Fuqua SA, Hilsenbeck SH, Chamness GC, Osborne CK.

J Clin Oncol 12: 647–649, 1994. What have we learned about risk factors for local recurrence after breast-conserving surgery and irradiation? Harris JR, Gelman R.

J Clin Oncol 12: 653–660, 1994. Risk factors in breast-conservation therapy. Borger J, Kemperman H, Hart A,

J Clin Oncol 12: 888–894, 1994. Relationship of patient age to pathologic features of the tumor and prognosis for patients with stage I or II breast cancer. Nixon AJ, Neuberg D, Hayes DF, Gelman R, Connolly JL, Schnitt S, Abner A, Recht A, Vicini F, Harris JR.

J Clin Oncol 13: 424–429, 1995. High complete remission rates with primary neoadjuvant infusional chemotherapy for large early breast cancer. Smith IE, Walsh G, Jones A, Prendiville J, Johnston S, Gusterson B, Ramage F, Robertshaw H, Sacks N, Ebbs S, et al.

J Clin Oncol 13: 547–552, 1995. Randomized trial of chemoendocrine therapy started before or after surgery for treatment of primary breast cancer. Powles TJ, Hickish TF, Makris A, Ashley SE, O'Brien ME, Tidy VA, Casey S, Nash AG, Sacks N, Cosgrove D, et al.

J Clin Oncol 13: 1129–1135, 1995. Elevated serum c-erbB-2 antigen levels and decreased response to hormone therapy of breast cancer. Leitzel K, Teramoto Y, Konrad K, Chinchilli VM, Volas G, Grossberg H, Harvey H, Demers L, Lipton A.

J Clin Oncol 13: 1152–1159, 1995. Paclitaxel as second and subsequent therapy for metastatic breast cancer: activity independent of prior anthracycline response. Seidman AD, Reichman BS, Crown JP, Yao TJ, Currie V, Hakes TB, Hudis CA, Gilewski TA, Baselga J, Forsythe P, et al.

J Clin Oncol 13: 2483–2489, 1995. High-dose chemotherapy with hematopoietic rescue as primary treatment for metastatic breast cancer: a randomized trial. Bezwoda WR, Seymour L, Dansey RD.

J Clin Oncol 13: 2722–2730, 1995. Intravenous vinorelbine as first-line and second-line therapy in advanced breast cancer. Weber BL, Vogel C, Jones S, Harvey H, Hutchins L, Bigley J, Hohneker J.

J Clin Oncol 13: 2731–2736, 1995. Advanced breast cancer: a phase II trial with gemcitabine. Carmichael J, Possinger K, Phillip P, Beykirch M, Kerr H, Walling J, Harris AL.

J Clin Oncol 13: 2869–2878, 1995. Adequate locoregional treatment for early breast cancer may prevent secondary dissemination. Arriagada R, Rutqvist LE, Mattsson A, Kramar A, Rotstein S.

J Clin Oncol 13: 2879–2885, 1995. Phase II trial of docetaxel in advanced thracycline-resistant or anthracenedione-resistant breast cancer. Ravdin PM, Burris HA, Cook G, Eisenberg P, Kane M, Bierman WA, Mortimer J, Genevois E, Bellet RE.

J Clin Oncol 13: 2886–2894, 1995. Phase II trial of docetaxel: a new, highly effective antineoplastic agent in the management of patients with anthracycline-resistant metastatic breast cancer. Valero V, Holmes FA, Walters RS, Theriault RL, Esparza L, Fraschini G, Fonseca GA, Bellet RE, Buzdar AU, Hortobagyi GN.

J Clin Oncol 14(1): 78–84, January 1996. Effect of tamoxifen on bone mineral density measured by dual-energy X-ray absorptiometry in healthy premenopausal and postmenopausal women. Powles TJ, Hickish T, Kanis JA, Tidy A, Ashley S.

J Clin Oncol 14: 737–744, 1996. Phase II study of weekly intravenous recombinant humanized anti-p185HER2 monoclonal antibody in patients with HER2/neu-overexpressing metastatic breast cancer. Baselga J, Tripathy D, Mendelsohn J, Baughman S, Benz C, Dantis L, Sklarin NT, Seidman AD, Hudis CA, Moore J, Rosen PP, Twaddell T, Henderson IC, Norton L.

J Clin Oncol 14: 754–763, 1996. Fifteen-year results of breast-conserving surgery and definitive breast irradiation for the treatment of ductal carcinoma in situ of the breast. Solin LJ, Kurtz J, Fourquet A, Amalric R, Recht A, Bornstein BA, Kuske R, Taylor M, Barrett W, Fowble B, Haffty B, Schultz DJ, Yeh IT, McCormick B, McNeese M.

J Clin Oncol 14(5): 1558–1564, 1996. Conservative treatment versus mastectomy in early breast cancer: patterns of failure with 15 years of follow-up data. Institut Gustave-Roussy Breast Cancer Group. Arriagada R, Le MG, Rochard F, Contesso G.

J Clin Oncol 14: 1858–1867, 1996. Multicenter, randomized comparative study of two doses of paclitaxel in patients with metastatic breast cancer. Nabholtz JM, Gelmon K, Bontenbal M, Spielmann M, Catimel G, Conte P, Klaassen U, Namer M, Bonneterre J, Fumoleau P, Winograd B.

J Clin Oncol 14: 1982–1992, 1996. Sequential methotrexate and fluorouracil for the treatment of node-negative breast cancer patients with estrogen receptor-negative tumors: eight-year results from National Surgical Adjuvant Breast and Bowel Project (NSABP) B-13 and first report of findings from NSABP B-19 comparing methotrexate and fluorouracil with conventional cyclophosphamide, methotrexate, and fluorouracil. Fisher B, Dignam J, Mamounas EP, Costantino JP, Wickerham DL, Redmond C, Wolmark N, Dimitrov NV, Bowman DM, Glass AG, Atkins JN, Abramson N, Sutherland CM, Aron BS, Margolese RG.

J Clin Oncol; 14(7): 2000–11, 1996. Anastrozole, a potent and selective aromatase inhibitor, versus megestrol acetate in postmenopausal women with advanced breast cancer: results of overview analysis of two phase III trials Arimidex Study Group. Buzdar A, Jonat W, Howell A, Jones SE, Blomqvist C, Vogel CL, Eiermann W, Wolter JM, Azab M, Webster A, Plourde PV.

J Clin Oncol 14(8): 2197–2205, 1996. Long-term follow-up of patients with complete remission following combination chemotherapy for metastatic breast cancer. Greenberg PA, Hortobagyi GN, Smith TL, Ziegler LD, Frye DK, Buzdar AU.

J Clin Oncol 14: 2552–2559, 1996. Delay in progression of bone metastases in breast cancer patients treated with intravenous pamidronate: results from a multinational randomized controlled trial: The Aredia Multinational Cooperative Group. Conte PF, Latreille J, Mauriac L, Calabresi F, Santos R, Campos D, Bonneterre J, Francini G, Ford JM.

J Clin Oncol 14: 2702–2708, 1996. c-erb B2 overexpression decreases the benefit of adjuvant tamoxifen in early-stage breast cancer without axillary lymph node metastases. Carlomagno C, Perrone F, Gallo C, De Laurentiis M, Lauria R, Morabito A, Pettinato G, Panico L, D'Antonio A, Bianco AR, De Placido S.

J Clin Oncol 14(10), 2713–2721, October 1996. Sequence-dependent alteration of doxorubicin pharmacokinetics by paclitaxel in a phase I study of paclitaxel and doxorubicin in patients with metastatic breast cancer. Holmes FA, Madden T, Newman RA, Valero V, Theriault RL, Fraschini G, Walters RS, Booser DJ, Buzdar AU, Willey J, Hortobagyi GN.

J Clin Oncol 14(10): 2722–2730, October 1996. Treatment-related leukemia in breast cancer patients treated with fluorouracil-doxorubicin-cyclophosphamide combination adjuvant chemotherapy: the University of Texas M.D. Anderson Cancer Center experience. Diamandidou E, Buzdar AU, Smith TL, Frye D, Witjaksono M, Hortobagyi GN.

J Clin Oncol 14: 2731–2737, 1996. Increased thromboembolic complications with concurrent tamoxifen and chemotherapy in a randomized trial of adjuvant therapy for women with breast cancer. National Cancer Institute of Canada Clinical Trials Group Breast Cancer Site Group. Pritchard KI, Paterson AH, Paul NA, Zee B, Fine S, Pater J.

J Clin Oncol 14(10): 2843–2877, 1996. Clinical practice guidelines for the use of tumor markers in breast and colorectal cancer. Adopted on May 17, 1996 by the American Society of Clinical Oncology.

J Clin Oncol 14(12): 3097–3104, 1996. Efficacy and tolerance of vinorelbine and fluorouracil combination as first-line chemotherapy of advanced breast cancer: results of a phase II study using a sequential group method. Dieras V, Extra JM, Bellissant E, Espie M, Morvan F, Pierga JY, Mignot L, Tresca P, Marty M.

J Clin Oncol 15: 963–968, 1997. Role of a 10-Gy boost in the conservative treatment of early breast cancer: results of a randomized clinical trial in Lyon, France. Romestaing P, Lehingue Y, Carrie C, Coquard R, Montbarbon X, Ardiet JM, Mamelle N, Gerard JP.

J Clin Oncol 15(4): 1385–1394. April 1997. Effectiveness of adjuvant chemotherapy in combination with tamoxifen for node-positive postmenopausal breast cancer patients. International Breast Cancer Study Group.

J Clin Oncol 15: 1870–1879, 1997. High-dose chemotherapy with autologous hematopoietic stem-cell support for breast cancer in North America. Antman KH, Rowlings PA, Vaughan WP, Pelz CJ, Fay JW, Fields KK, Freytes CO, Gale RP, Hillner BE, Holland HK, Kennedy MJ, Klein JP, Lazarus HM, McCarthy PL, Saez R, Spitzer G, Stadtmauer EA, Williams SF, Wolff S, Sobocinski KA, Armitage JO, Horowitz MM.

J Clin Oncol 15(5): 1906–1915, May 1997. Human pharmacokinetic characterization and in vitro study of the interaction between doxorubicin and paclitaxel in patients with breast cancer. Gianni L, Vigano L, Locatelli A, Capri G, Giani A, Tarenzi E, Bonadonna G.

J Clin Oncol 15(5): 2149–2156, 1997. Recommended breast cancer surveillance guidelines American Society of Clinical Oncology, Adopted February 20, 1997.

J Clin Oncol 15(7): 2483–2493, 1997. Effect of preoperative chemotherapy on local-regional disease in women with operable breast cancer: findings from National Surgical Adjuvant Breast and Bowel Project B-18. Fisher B, Brown A, Mamounas E, Wieand S, Robidoux A, Margolese RG, Cruz AB Jr, Fisher ER, Wickerham DL, Wolmark N, DeCillis A, Hoehn JL, Lees AW, Dimitrov NV.

J Clin Oncol 16(2): 441–452, 1998. Lumpectomy and radiation therapy for the treatment of intraductal breast cancer: findings from National Surgical Adjuvant Breast and Bowel Project B-17. Fisher B, Dignam J, Wolmark N, Mamounas E, Costantino J, Poller W, Fisher ER, Wickerham DL, Deutsch M, Margolese R, Dimitrov N, Kavanah M.

J Clin Oncol 16(2): 453–461, 1998. Letrozole, a new oral aromatase inhibitor for advanced breast cancer: double-blind randomized trial showing a dose effect and improved efficacy and tolerability compared with megestrol acetate. Dombernowsky P, Smith I, Falkson G, Leonard R, Panasci L, Bellmunt J, Bezwoda W, Gardin G, Gudgeon A, Morgan M, Fornasiero A, Hoffmann W, Michel J, Hatschek T, Tjabbes T, Chaudri HA, Hornberger U, Trunet PF.

J Clin Oncol 16(2): 495–500, 1998. Prospective evaluation of vitamin E for hot flashes in breast cancer survivors. Barton DL, Loprinzi CL, Quella SK, Sloan JA, Veeder MH, Egner JR, Fidler P, Stella PJ, Swan DK, Vaught NL, Novotny P.

J Clin Oncol 16(3): 1008–1012, 1998. Secondary myelodysplasia and acute leukemia in breast cancer patients after autologous bone marrow transplant. Laughlin MJ, McGaughey DS, Crews JR, Chao NJ, Rizzieri D, Ross M, Gockerman J, Cirrincione C, Berry D, Mills L, Defusco P, LeGrand S, Peters WP, Vredenburgh JJ.

J Clin Oncol 16(6): 2038–2044, 1998. Long-term prevention of skeletal complications of metastatic breast cancer with pamidronate. Protocol 19 Aredia Breast Cancer Study Group. Hortobagyi GN, Theriault RL, Lipton A, Porter L, Blayney D, Sinoff C, Wheeler H, Simeone JF, Seaman JJ, Knight RD, Heffernan M, Mellars K, Reitsma DJ.

J Clin Oncol 16(8)Aug;16(8): 2651–2658, 1998. Randomized trial of intensive cyclophosphamide, epirubicin, and fluorouracil chemotherapy compared with cyclophosphamide, methotrexate, and fluorouracil in premenopausal women with node-positive breast cancer. National Cancer Institute of Canada Clinical Trials Group. Levine MN, Bramwell VH, Pritchard KI, Norris BD, Shepherd LE, Abu-Zahra H, Findlay B, Warr D, Bowman D, Myles J, Arnold A, Vandenberg T, MacKenzie R, Robert J, Ottaway J, Burnell M, Williams CK, Tu D.

J Epidemiol Community Health; 50(3): 353–8, 1996. Long term breast cancer screening in Nijmegen, The Netherlands: the nine rounds from 1975–1992. Otten JD, van Dijck JA, Peer PG, Straatman H, Verbeek AL, Mravunac M, Hendriks JH, Holland R.

J Hematother 5(1): 57–62, February 1996. A comparison of immunohistochemistry, two-color immuno-fluorescence, and flow cytometry with cell sorting for the detection of micrometastatic breastcancer in the bone marrow. Vredenburgh JJ, Silva O, Tyer C, DeSombre K, Abou-Ghalia A, Cook M, Layfield L, Peters WP, Bast RC, Jr.

J Hematother 5: 519–24, 1996. Micrometastases and transplantation. Sharp JG.

J Natl Cancer Inst 48: 605–613, 1972. Menopause and breast cancer risk. Trichopoulos D, MacMahon B, Cole P.

J Natl Cancer Inst 69(2): 349–355, 1982. Ten- to fourteen-year effect of screening on breast cancer mortality. Shapiro S, Venet W, Strax P, Venet L, Roeser R.

J Natl Cancer Inst 83(13): 920–926, 1991. High-dose chemotherapy with reinfusion of purged autologous bone marrow following dose-intense induction as initial therapy for metastatic breast cancer. Kennedy MJ, Beveridge RA, Rowley SD, Gordon GB, Abeloff MD, Davidson NE.

J Natl Cancer Inst 83: 1299–1306, 1991. Contralateral primary tumors in breast cancer patients in a randomized trial of adjuvant tamoxifen therapy. Rutqvist LE, Cedermark B, Glas U, Mattsson A, Skoog L, Somell A, Theve T, Wilking N, Skergren J, Hjalmar ML, et al.

J Natl Cancer Inst 85: 1644–1656, 1993. Report of the International Workshop on Screening for Breast Cancer. Fetcher SW, Black W, Harris R, Rimer BK, Shapiro S.

J Natl Cancer Inst 86(7): 527–537, 1994. Endometrial cancer in tamoxifen-treated breast cancer patients: findings from the National Surgical Adjuvant Breast and Bowel Project, NSABP B-14. Fisher B, Costantino JP, Redmond CK, Fisher ER, Wickerham DL, Cronin WM.

J Natl Cancer Inst 86: 705–712, 1994. Tumor biologic factors and breast cancer prognosis among white, Hispanic, and black women in the United States. Elledge RM, Clark GM, Chamness GC, Osborne CK.

J Natl Cancer Inst 86: 1403–1408, 1994. Physical exercise and reduced risk of breast cancer in young women. Bernstein L, Henderson BE, Hanisch R, Sullivan-Halley J, Ross RK.

J Natl Cancer Inst 86: 1534–1539, 1994. Effects of tamoxifen on cardiovascular risk factors in postmenopausal women after 5 years of treatment. Love RR, Wiebe DA, Feyzi JM, Newcomb PA, Chappell RJ.

J Natl Cancer Inst 87(1): 19-27, 1995. Local recurrences and distant metastases after conservative breast cancer treatments: partly independent events. Veronesi U, Marubini E, Del Vecchio M, Manzari A, Andreola S, Greco M, Luini A, Merson M, Saccozzi R, Rilke F, et al.

J Natl Cancer Inst 87(9): 645–651, 1995. Adjuvant tamoxifen therapy for early stage breast cancer and second primary malignancies. Stockholm Breast Cancer Study Group. Rutqvist LE, Johansson H, Signomklao T, Johansson U, Fornander T, Wilking N.

J Natl Cancer Inst 87: 1829, 1995. NSABP halts B-14 trial: no benefit seen beyond 5 years of tamoxifen use. No Authors given.

J Natl Cancer Inst 88(21): 1529–1542, 1996. Five versus more than five years of tamoxifen therapy for breast cancer patients with negative lymph nodes and estrogen receptor-positive tumors. Fisher B, Dignam J, Bryant J, DeCillis A, Wickerham DL, Wolmark N, Costantino J, Redmond C, Fisher ER, Bowman DM, Deschenes L, Dimitrov NV, Margolese RG, Robidoux A, Shibata H, Terz J, Paterson AH, Feldman MI, Farrar W, Evans J, Lickley HL.

J Natl Cancer Inst; 88(22): 1652–8, 1996. Micrometastatic breast cancer cells in bone marrow at primary surgery: prognostic value in comparison with nodal status. Diel IJ, Kaufmann M, Costa SD, Holle R, von Minckwitz G, Solomayer EF, Kaul S, Bastert G.

J Natl Cancer Inst 88: 1659–1664, 1996. Randomized clinical trials of breast irradiation following lumpectomy and axillary dissection for node negative breast cancer: An Update. Clark RM, Whelan T, Levine M, Roberts R, Willan A, McCulloch P, Lipa M, Wilkinson RH, Mahoney LJ.

J Natl Cancer Inst 88: 1828–1833, 1996. Postchemotherapy adjuvant tamoxifen therapy beyond five years in patients with lymph node-positive breast cancer. Eastern Cooperative Oncology Group. Tormey DC, Gray R, Falkson HC.

J Natl Cancer Inst 89(22): 1652–1654, 1997. Adjuvant therapy for early breast cancer: a time to refine. Powles TJ.

J Natl Cancer Inst 90(3): 210–218, 1998. Impairment of cognitive function in women receiving adjuvant treatment for high-risk breast cancer: high-dose versus standard-dose chemotherapy. van Dam FS, Schagen SB, Muller MJ, Boogerd W, v d Wall E, Droogleever Fortuyn ME, Rodenhuis S.

J Natl Cancer Inst 90(15):1155–1160, 1998. Physical activity and breast cancer risk in a cohort of young women. Rockhill B, Willett WC, Hunter DJ, Manson JE, Hankinson SE, Spiegelman D, Colditz GA.

J Natl Cancer Inst 90(16):1205–1211, 1998. Dose and dose intensity as determinants of outcome in the adjuvant treatment of breast cancer. The Cancer and Leukemia Group B. Budman DR, Berry DA, Cirrincione CT, Henderson IC, Wood WC, Weiss RB, Ferree CR, Muss HB, Green MR, Norton L, Frei E 3rd.

JNCI Monogr 1: 55–70, 1986. Adjuvant treatment for early breast cancer: the Ludwig breast cancer studies. Goldhirsch A, Gelber R.

JNCI Monogr 11: 7–13, 1992. Lumpectomy for breast cancer: an update of the NSABP experience. National Surgical Adjuvant Breast and Bowel Project. Fisher B, Redmond C.

JNCI Monogr 11: 15–18, 1992. Randomized clinical trial to assess the value of breast-conserving therapy in stage I and II breast cancer-EORTC 10801 Trial. VanDongen JA, Bartelink H, Fentiman T, Lerut T, Mignolet F.

JNCI Monog 11: 19–25, 1992. Danish randomized trial comparing breast cancer conservation therapy with mastectomy: Six year of life-table analysis. Blichert-Toft M, Rose C, Andersen JA, Overgaard M.

JNCI Monogr 11: 33–39, 1992. Recurrence in the breast following conservative surgery and radiation therapy for early-stage breast cancer. Vicini FA, Recht A, Abner A, Boyages J, Cady B, Connolly JL, Gelman R, Osteen RT, Schnitt SJ, Silen W, et al.

JNCI Monogr 11: 41–48, 1992. Surgical consideration in selecting local therapy. Margolese R.

JNCI Monogr 11: 105–116, 1992. Systemic therapy in node-negative patients: updated findings from NSABP clinical trials National Surgical Adjuvant Breast and Bowel Project. Fisher B, Redmond C.

JNCI Monogr 11: 117–120, 1992. The Scottish trial of adjuvant tamoxifen in node-negative breast cancer. Stewart HJ.

JNCI Monogr 11: 151–158, 1992. Prognostic factors in NSABP studies of women with node-negative breast cancer National Surgical Adjuvant Breast and Bowel Project. Fisher ER, Redmond C, Fisher B.

JNCI Monogr 16:35–42, 1994. Breast cancer outcome and predictors of outcome: are there age differentials? Albain KS, Allred DC, Clark GM.

JNCI Monogr, 19: 41–4, 1995. Randomized, comparative study of high-dose, with autologous bone marrow support versus low-dose cyclophosphamide, cisplatin, and carmustine as consolidation to adjuvant cyclophosphamide, doxorubicin, and fluorouracil for patients with operable stage II or III breast cancer involving 10 or more axillary lymph nodes, CALGB Protocol 9082) Cancer and Leukemia Group B. Hurd DD, Peters WP.

J Pathol 175: 195–201, 1995. Loss of heterozygosity in ductal carcinoma in situ of the breast. Stratton M, Collins N, Lakhani S, Sloane J.

J Surg Oncol 47: 139–147, 1991. Conservative management of intraductal carcinoma, DCIS) of the breast Collaborating NSABP investigators. Fisher ER, Leeming R, Anderson S, Redmond C, Fisher B.

J Surg Oncol 48: 260–267, 1991. p53 alterations in all stages of breast cancer. Davidoff AM, Kerns BJ, Pence JC, Marks JR, Iglehart JD.

J Surg Oncol 64(1): 27–31, January 1997. Seroma formation following axillary dissection for breast cancer: risk factors and lack of influence of bovine thrombin. Burak WE Jr, Goodman PS, Young DC, Farrar WB.

J Am Med Assoc 265: 391–395, 1991. NIH consensus conference Treatment of early-stage breast cancer, (no author given).

J Am Med Assoc 268: 2037–2044, 1992. Dietary fat and fiber in relation to risk of breast cancer An 8-year follow-up. Willett WC, Hunter DJ, Stampfer MJ, Colditz G, Manson JE, Spiegelman D, Rosner B, Hennekens CH, Speizer FE.

J Am Med Assoc 275: 283–287, 1996. Pregnancy termination in relation to risk of breast cancer. Newcomb PA, Storer BE, Longnecker MP, Mittendorf R, Greenberg ER, Willett WC.

J Am Med Assoc 278: 1407–1411, 1997. Dual effects of weight and weight gain on breast cancer risk. Huang Z, Hankinson SE, Colditz GA, Stampfer MJ, Hunter DJ, Manson JE, Hennekens CH, Rosner B, Speizer FE, Willett WC.

J Am Med Assoc 279: 688–695, 1998. Estrogen therapy in postmenopausal women, effects on cognitive function and dementia. Yaffe K, Sawaya G, Lieberburg I, Grady D.

Lancet 30: 435–438, 30 August. Intra-arterial chemotherapy as basal treatment in advanced and fungating primary breast cancer. Stephens FO, Crea P, Harker GJS, Roberts BA, Hambly CK.

Lancet 2: 171–172, 1983. Failure of chloroquine prophylaxis in Plasmodium falciparum in Zaire. Moran JS.

Lancet 2(8608): 411–416, 20 Augsut 1988. First results on mortality reduction in the UK Trial of Early Detection of Breast Cancer UK Trial of Early Detection of Breast Cancer Group.

Lancet 335: 186–190, 1990. Comparison of short-term and continuous chemotherapy, mitozantrone) for advanced breast cancer. Harris AL, Mcantwell B, Carmichael J, Wilson R, Farndon J, Dawes P, Ghani S, Evans RG.

Lancet 335(8688): 519–522, 1990. Extent, distribution, and mammographic/histological correlations of breast ductal carcinoma in situ. Holland R, Hendriks JH, Vebeek AL, Mravunac M, Schuurmans Stekhoven JH.

Lancet 337: 1197–1200, 1991. Dietary effects on breast-cancer risk in Singapore. Lee HP, Gourley L, Duffy SW, Esteve J, Lee J, Day NE.

Lancet 339: 1–15, 1992. Systemic treatment of early breast cancer by hormonal, cytotoxic, or immune therapy 133 randomised trials involving 31000 recurrences and 24000 deaths among 75000 women Early Breast Cancer Trialists' Collaborative Group.

Lancet 339: 71–85, 1992. Systemic treatment of early breast cancer by hormonal, cytotoxic, or immune therapy Early Breast Cancer Trialists Collaborative Group.

Lancet 339(8790): 412–414, 1992. Breast cancer treatment and natural history: new insights from results of screening. Tabar L, Fagerberg G, Day NE, Duffy SW, Kitchin RM.

Lancet 341: 1293–1298, 1993. Adjuvant ovarian ablation versus CMF chemotherapy in premenopausal women with pathological stage II breast carcinoma: the Scottish trial Scottish Cancer Trials Breast Group and ICRF Breast Unit, Guy's Hospital, London.

Lancet 341: 1485, 1993. Preoperative chemotherapy in operable breast cancer. Bonadonna G, Valagussa P, Brambilla C, Ferrari L.

Lancet 343: 692–695, 1994. Risks of cancer in BRCA1-mutation carriers Breast Cancer Linkage Consortium. Ford D, Easton DF, Bishop DT, Narod SA, Goldgar DE.

Lancet 343: 1587–1589, 1994. Effect of pregnancy on prognosis for young women with breast cancer. Guinee VF, Olsson H, Moller T, Hess KR, Taylor SH, Fahey T, Gladikov JV, van den Blink JW, Bonichon F, Dische S, et al.

Lancet 345(8958): 1181–1182, 1995. p53 protein overexpression and chemosensitivity in breast cancer. Makris A, Powles TJ, Dowsett M, Allred C.

Lancet 347: 1713–1727, 1996. Collaborative Group on Hormonal Factors in Breast Cancer: Breast cancer and hormonal contraceptives: collaborative reanalysis of individual data on 53297 ♀ with breast cancer and 100239 ♀ without breast cancer from 54 epidemiologic studies.

Lancet 348: 708–713, 1996. Randomized controlled trial of conservation therapy for breast cancer: Six year analysis of the Scottish Trial. Forrest AP, Steward HJ, Everington D, Prescott RJ, Mcardle CS, Harnett AN, Smith DC, George WD.

Lancet 348(9036): 1189–1196, 1996. EBCTCG Ovarian ablation in early breast cancer: Overview of the randomized trials.

Lancet 350(9083): 990–994, 4 October 1997. Case-control study of phyto-oestrogens and breast cancer Ingram D, Sanders K, Kolybaba M, Lopez D.

Lancet 349: 1864–1867, 1997. Sentinel-node biopsy to avoid axillary dissection in breast cancer with clinically negative lymph-nodes. Veronesi U, Paganelli G, Galimberti V, Viale G, Zurrida S, Bedoni M, Costa A, de Cicco C, Geraghty JG, Luini A, Sacchini V, Veronesi P.

Lancet 351: 316–321, 1998. Survival and tumour characteristics of breast cancer patients with germline mutations of BRCA1. Verhoog LC, Beckelmans CTM, Seynaeve C, van den Bosch LMC, Dahmen G.

Lancet 352: 93–97, 1998. Prevention of breast cancer with tamoxifen: preliminary findings from the Italian randomised trial among hysterectomised women. Itali an Tamoxifen Prevention Study. Veronesi U, Maisonneuve P, Costa A, Sacchini V, Maltoni C, Robertson C, Rotmensz N, Boyle P.

Mayo Clin Proc 67: 128–130, 1992. Hemorrhagic cystitis complicating bone marrow transplantation. Lettendre L, Hoagland HC, Gertz MA.

Menopause 2: 73–80, 1995. Current opinion: hormone replacement therapy after a diagnosis of breast cancer. Sands R, Boshoff C, Jones A, et al.

Nat Genet 8: 105–106, 1994. The glittering prize. No author named.

Nat Genet 13: 114–116, 1996. Localization of the gene for Cowden's disease to chromosome 10q22-23. Nelen MR, Padberg GW, Peeters EA, Lin AY, van den Helm B, Frants RR, et al.

Nat Genet 13: 117–119, 1996. A single BRCA2 mutation in male and female breast cancer families from Iceland with varied cancer phenotypes. Thorlacius S, Olafsdottir G, Tryggvadottir L, Neuhausen S, Jonasson JG, Tavpigian SV, et al.

Nat Genet 13: 126–128, 1996. Recurrent BRCA2 6174delT mutations in Ashkenazi Jewish women affected by breast cancer. Neuhausen S, Gilwski T, Norton L, Tran T, McGuire P, Swensen J, et al.

Neurology 39: 502–506, 1989. Distinction between neoplastic and radiation-induced brachial plexopathy, with emphasis on the role of EMG. Harper CM, Thomas JE, Cascino TL, Litchy WJ.

New Engl J Med 292: 117–122, 1975. 1-Phenylalanine mustard, L-PAM) in the management of primary breast cancer A report of early findings. Fisher B, Carbone P, Economou SG, Frelick R, Glass A, Lerner H, Redmond C, Zelen M, Band P, Katrych DL, Wolmark N, Fisher ER.

New Engl J Med 309: 1094–1104, 1983. The pharmacology and clinical use of methotrexate. Jolivet J, Cowan KH, Curt GA, Clendeninn NJ, Chabner BA.

New Engl J Med 312: 146–151, 1985. Risk factors for breast cancer in women with proliferative breast disease. Dupont WD, Page DL.

New Engl J Med 312: 674–681, 1985. Ten-year results of a randomized clinical trial comparing radical mastectomy and total mastectomy with or without radiation. Fisher B, Redmond C, Fisher ER, Bauer M, Wolmark N, Wickerham DL, Deutsch M, Montague E, Margolese R, Foster R.

New Engl J Med 316: 1174–1180, 1987. Moderate alcohol consumption and the risk of breast cancer. Willett WC, Stampfer MJ, Colditz GA, Rosner BA, Hennekens CH, Speizer FE.

New Engl J Med 317: 1490–1495, 1987. Improving the quality of life during chemotherapy for advanced breast cancer A comparison of intermittent and continuous treatment strategies. Coates A, Gebski V, Bishop JF, Jeal PN, Woods RL, Snyder R, Tattersall MH, Byrne M, Harvey V, Gill G.

New Engl J Med 319: 677–683, 1988. Combination adjuvant chemotherapy for node-positive breast cancer: Inadequacy of a single perioperative cycle. The Ludwig Breast Cancer Study Group.

New Engl J Med 319: 1239–1245, 1988. Neu-protein overexpression in breast cancer Association with comedo-type ductal carcinoma in situ and limited prognostic value in stage II breast cancer. van de Vijver MJ, Peterse JL, Mooi WJ, Wisman P, Lomans J, Dalesio O, Nusse R.

New Engl J Med 320: 473–478, 1989. A randomized clinical trial evaluating sequential methotrexate and fluorouracil in the treatment of patients with node-negative breast cancer who have estrogen-receptor-negative tumors. Fisher B, Redmond C, Dimitrov NV, Bowman D, Legault-Poisson S, Wickerham, Wolmark N, Fisher ER, Margolese R, Sutherland C.

New Engl J Med 320: 822–828, 1989. Eight-year results of a randomized clinical trial comparing total mastectomy and lumpectomy with or without irradiation in the treatment of breast cancer. Fisher B, Redmond C, Poisson R, Margolese R, Wolmark N, Wickerham L, Fisher E, Deutsch M, Caplan R, Pilch Y, et al.

New Engl J Med 321: 293–297, 1989. The risk of breast cancer after estrogen and estrogen-progestin replacement. Bergkvist L, Adami HO, Persson I, Hoover R, Schairer C.

New Engl J Med 322: 494–500, 1990. A randomized trial of surgery in the treatment of single metastases to the brain. Patchell RA, Tibbs PA, Walsh JW, Dempsey RJ, Maruyama Y, Kryscio RJ, Markesbery WJ, Macdonald JS, Young B.

New Engl J Med 325: 1342–1348, 1991. Interrupted versus continuous chemotherapy in patients with metastatic breast cancer The Piedmont Oncology Association. Muss HB, Case LD, Richards F, White DR, Cooper MR, Cruz JM, Powell BL, Spurr CL, Capizzi RL.

New Engl J Med 325: 1831–1836, 1991. Incidence of cancer in 161 families affected by ataxia-telangiectasia. Swift M, Morrell D, Massey RB, Chase CL.

New Engl J Med 326: 713–714, 1992. Physicians and occupational medicine. Markowitz S, Frank AL, Hessl SM, Christiani D, Robins T, Balmes J.

New Engl J Med 326: 852–856, 1992. Effects of tamoxifen on bone mineral density in postmenopausal women with breast cancer. Love RR, Mazess RB, Barden HS, Epstein S, Newcomb PA, Jordan VC, Carbone PP, DeMets DL.

New Engl J Med 326: 1745–1751, 1992. Risk of leukemia after chemotherapy and radiation treatment for breast cancer. Curtis RE, Boice JD, Stovall M, Bernstein L, Greenberg RS, Flannery JT, Schwartz AG, Weyer P, Moloney WC, Hoover RN.

New Engl J Med; 326(26): 1756–61, 1992. Prognostic factors and treatment decisions in axillary-node-negative breast cancer. McGuire WL, Clark GM.

New Engl J Med 327: 319–328, 1992. Breast cancer, 1) Harris JR, Lippman ME, Veronesi U, Willett W.

New Engl J Med 327: 390–398, 1992. Breast cancer, 2) Harris JR, Lippman ME, Veronesi U, Willett W.

New Engl J Med 327: 937–942, 1992. Evaluation of a palpable breast mass. Donegan WL.

New Engl J Med 328: 1581–1586, 1993. Lumpectomy compared with lumpectomy and radiation therapy for the treatment of intraductal breast cancer. Fisher B, Costantino J, Redmond C, Fisher E, Margolese R, Dimitrov N, Wolmark N, Wickerham DL, Deutsch M, Ore L, et al.

New Engl J Med 328: 1587–1591, 1993. Radiotherapy after breast-preserving surgery in women with localized cancer of the breast. Veronesi U, Luini A, Del Vecchio M, Greco M, Galimberti V, Merson M, Rilke F, Sacchini V, Saccozzi R, Savio T, et al.

New Engl J Med 329: 234–240, 1993. A prospective study of the intake of vitamins C, E, and A and the risk of breast cancer. Hunter DJ, Manson JE, Colditz GA, Stampfer MJ, Rosner B, Hennekens CH, Speizer FE, Willett WC.

New Engl J Med 330: 81–87, 1994. Lactation and a reduced risk of premenopausal breast cancer. Newcomb PA, Storer BE, Longnecker MP, Mittendorf R, Greenberg ER, Clapp RW, Burke KP, Willett WC, MacMahon B.

New Engl J Med 330: 473–477, 1994. Variation in approval by insurance companies of coverage for autologous bone marrow transplantation for breast cancer. Peters WP, Rogers MC.

New Engl J Med 330: 1253–1259, 1994. Dose and dose intensity of adjuvant chemotherapy for stage II, node-positive breast carcinoma. Wood WC, Budman DR, Korzun AH, Cooper MR, Younger J, Hart RD, Moore A, Ellerton JA, Norton L, Ferree CR, et al.

New Engl J Med 330: 1260–1266, 1994. c-erbB-2 expression and response to adjuvant therapy in women with node-positive early breast cancer. Muss HB, Thor AD, Berry DA, Kute T, Liu ET, Koerner F, Cirrincione CT, Budman DR, Wood WC, Barcos M, et al.

New Engl J Med 330: 1683, 1994. Breast-feeding and breast cancer. Ross RK, Yu MC.

New Engl J Med 331: 5–9, 1994. Transient increases in the risk of breast cancer after giving birth. Lambe M, Hseih C, Trichopoulos D, Ekbom A, Pavia M, Adami HO.

New Engl J Med 331: 10–15, 1994. Long-term risk of breast cancer in women with fibroadenoma. Dupont, WD, Page, DL, Parl FF, Vnencak-Jones CL, Plummer WD, Rados MS, Schuyler PA.

New Engl J Med 331: 347–52, 1994. Megestrol acetate for the prevention of hot flashes. Loprinzi CL, Midlak JC, Quella SK, O'Fallon JR, Hatfield AK, Nelimark RA, Dose AM, Fischer T, Johnson C, Klatt NE, et al.

New Engl J Med 332: 901–906, 1995. Adjuvant cyclophosphamide, methotrexate, and fluorouracil in node-positive breast cancer: the results of 20 years of follow-up. Bonadonna G, Valagussa P, Moliterni A, Zambetti M, Brambilla C.

New Engl J Med 332: 907–911, 1995. Ten-year results of a comparison of conservation with mastectomy in the treatment of stage I and II breast cancer. Jacobson JA, Danforth DN, Cowan KH, d'Angelo T, Steinberg SM, Pierce L, Lippman ME, Lichter AS, Glatstein E, Okunieff P.

New Engl J Med 332: 1589–1593, 1995. The use of estrogens and progestins and the risk of breast cancer in postmenopausal women. Colditz GA, Hankinson SE, Hunter DJ, Willett WC, Manson JE, Stampfer MJ, Hennekens C, Rosner B, Speizer FE.

New Engl J Med 333: 1444–1455, 1995. Effects of radiotherapy and surgery in early breast cancer An overview of the randomized trials Early Breast Cancer Trialists' Collaborative Group.

New Engl J Med 333: 1456–1461, 1995. Reanalysis and results after 12 years of follow-up in a randomized clinical trial comparing total mastectomy with lumpectomy with or without irradiation in the treatment of breast cancer. Fisher B, Anderson S, Redmond CK, Wolmark N, Wickerham DL, Cronin WM.

New Engl J Med 333: 1757–1763, 1995. Seminars in Medicine of the Beth Israel Hospital, Boston Clinical applications of research on angiogenesis. Folkman J.

New Engl J Med 334: 137–142, 1996. BRCA1 mutations in a population-based sample of young women with breast cancer. Langston AA, Malone KE, Thompson JD, Daling JR, Ostrander EA.

New Engl J Med 334: 143–149, 1996. Germ-line BRCA1 mutations in Jewish and non-Jewish women with early-onset breast cancer. FitzGerald MG, MacDonald DJ, Krainer M, Hoover I, O'Neil E, Unsal H, Silva-Arrieto S, Finkelstein DM, Beer-Romero P, Englert C, Sgroi DC, Smith BL, Younger JW, Garber JE, Duda RB, Mayzel KA, Isselbacher KJ, Friend SH, Haber DA.

New Engl J Med 334: 356–361, 1996. Cohort studies of fat intake and the risk of breast cancer—a pooled analysis. Hunter DJ, Spiegelman D, Adami HO, Beeson L, van den Brandt PA, Folsom AR, Fraser GE, Goldbohm RA, Graham S, Howe GR, et al.

New Engl J Med 334: 745–751, 1996. Breast cancer and other second neoplasms after childhood Hodgkin's disease. Bhatia S, Robison LL, Oberlin O, Greenberg M, Bunin G, Fossati-Bellani F, Meadows AT.

New Engl J Med 334: 1356–1361, 1996. The sequencing of chemotherapy and radiation therapy after conservative surgery for early-stage breast cancer. Recht A, Come SE, Henderson IC, Gelman RS, Silver B, Hayes DF, Shulman LN, Harris JR.

Engl J Med 335: 1413–1416, 1996. Clinical and pathological features of ovarian cancer in women with germ-line mutations of BRCA1. Rubin SC, Benjamin I, Behbakht K, Takahashi H, Morgan MA, LiVolsi VA, Berchuck A, Muto MG, Garber JE, Weber BL, Lynch HT, Boyd J.

New Engl J Med 335: 1785–1791, 1996. Efficacy of pamidronate in reducing skeletal complications in patients with breast cancer and lytic bone metastases Protocol 19 Aredia Breast Cancer Study Group. Hortobagyi GN, Theriault RL, Porter L, Blayney D, Lipton A, Sinoff C, Wheeler H, Simeone JF, Seaman J, Knight RD.

New Engl J Med 336: 81–85, 1997. Induced abortion and the risk of breast cancer. Melbye M, Wohlfahrt J, Olsen, Frisch M, Westergaard T, Helweg-Larsen K, Andersen PK.

New Engl J Med 336: 677–682, 1997. Complications leading to surgery after breast implantation. Gabriel SE, Woods JE, O'Fallon WM, Beard CM, Kurland LT, Melton LJ.

New Engl J Med 336: 1269–1275, 1997. Physical activity and the risk of breast cancer. Thune I, Brenn T, Lund E, Gaard M.

New Engl J Med 336: 1401–1408, 1997. The risk of cancer associated with specific mutations of BRCA1 and BRCA2 among Ashkenazi Jews. Struewing JP, Hartge P, Wacholder S, Baker SM, Berlin M, McAdams M, Timmerman MM, Brody LC, Tucker MA.

New Engl J Med 336: 1416–1421, 1997. Differential contributions of BRCA1 and BRCA2 to early-onset breast cancer. Krainer M, Silva-Arrieta S, FitzGerald MG, Shimada A, Ishioka C, Kanamaru R, MacDonald DJ, Unsal H, Finkelstein DM, Bowcock A, Isselbacher KJ, Haber DA.

New Engl J Med 336(20): 1465–1471, 15 May 1997. Decision analysis—effects of prophylactic mastectomy and oophorectomy on life expectancy among women with BRCA1 or BRCA2 mutations. Schrag D, Kuntz KM, Garber JE, Weeks JC.

New Engl J Med 337: 949–955, 1997. Postoperative Radiotherapy in High-Risk Premenopausal Women with Breast Cancer Who Receive Adjuvant Chemotherapy. Overgaard M, Hansen PS, Overgaard J, Rose C, Andersson M, Bach F, Kjaer M, Gadeberg CC, Mouridsen HT, Jensen MB, Zedeler K.

New Engl J Med 337: 956–962, 1997. Adjuvant radiotherapy and chemotherapy in node-positive premenopausal women with breast cancer. Ragaz J, Jackson SM, Le N, Plenderleith IH, Spinelli JJ, Basco VE, Wilson KS, Knowling MA, Coppin CM, Paradis M, Coldman AJ, Olivotto IA.

New Engl J Med 337: 1253–1258, 1997. Plasma organochlorine levels and the risk of breast cancer. Hunter DJ, Hankinson SE, Laden F, Colditz GA, Manson JE, Willett WC, Speizer FE, Wolff MS.

New Engl J Med 337(23): 1641–1647, 4 December 1997. Effects of raloxifene on bone mineral density, serum cholesterol concentrations, and uterine endometrium in postmenopausal women. Delmas PD, Bjarnason NH, Mitlak BH, Ravoux AC, Shah AS, Huster WJ, Draper M, Christiansen C.

N Engl J Med 339(6): 357–363, 1998. Reduction in new metastases in breast cancer with adjuvant clodronate treatment. Diel IJ, Solomayer EF, Costa SD, Gollan C, Goerner R, Wallwiener D, Kaufmann M, Bastert G.

Nutr Cancer 12: 61–68, 1989. Fish consumption and breast cancer risk: An ecological study. Kaizer L, Boyd NF, Kriskov V, Tritchler D.

Nutr Cancer 12: 327–32, 1989. Estradiol binding to plasma proteins, after changing to a low-fat diet. Ingram D, Bennett F, Wood A.

Oncology 48: 265–269, 1991. Mitoxantrone as second-line single agent in metastatic breast cancer. Stein M, Borovik R, Robinson E.

Oncology 50: 222–225, 1993. Life long menstrual pattern and risk of breast cancer. Parazzini F, LaVecchia C, Negri E, Franceschi S, Tozzi L.

Oncology 8: 21–26, 1994. The role of excision and surveillance alone in subclinical DCIS of the breast. Schwartz GF.

Oncology(Huntington) 8(8): 25–31; discussion 35–36, 39–42, 1994. Detection and management of bone marrow micrometastases in breast cancer. Osborne MP, Rosen PP.

Oncology 51: 47–51, 1994. Immunohistochemical study on the expression of C-erbB-2 oncoprotein in breast cancer. Horiguchi J, Iino Y, Takei H, Yokoe T, Ishida T, Morishita Y.

Oncology, Huntingt; 9(8): 722, 1995. New lymphatic mapping may avoid many axillary dissectionsAnonymous.

Oncology 9: 756–60, 1995. Diagnosis and management of brachial plexus lesions in cancer patients. Kori SH.

Oncology 9: 767–73, 1995. Current status of vinorelbine for breast cancer. Smith GA.

Oncology, Huntingt 9(9): 877–886, September 1995. Current status of endocrine therapy for metastatic breast cancer. Kimmick G, Muss HB.

Oncology 10: 991–1002, 1996. Defining the role of post-mastectomy radiotherapy: the new evidence. Pierce LJ, Lichter A.

Oncology, Huntingt 11(5 Suppl 4): 23–28, May 1997. Phase III trials of toremifene vs. tamoxifen. Gams R.

Oncology, Huntingt; 11(5 Suppl 4): 29–36, 1997. High-dose toremifene vs. tamoxifen in postmenopausal advanced breast cancer. Gershanovich M, Hayes DF, Ellmen J, Vuorinen J.

Oncology 11(10): 1491–1501, 1997. Estrogen replacement therapy for breast cancer patients. Colditz GA.

Oncology 11: 213–239, 1997. Postmastectomy radiation: then and now. Fowble B.

Oncology 11, (suppl): 11–14, 1997. Docetaxel: today's results and tomorrow's promises. Hortobagyi GN.

Oncology 11, (suppl): 19–24, 1997. Docetaxel vs. doxorubicin in metastatic breast cancer resistant to alkylating chemotherapy. Chan S.

Oncology 11, (suppl): 15–18, 1997. Docetaxel as neoadjuvant chemotherapy in patients with stage III breast cancer. Gradisher WJ.

Oncology 11, (suppl 9): 9–17, 1997. Management of locally advanced breast cancer. Perez EA, Foo ML, Fulmer JT.

Oncology, Huntingt; 11(11A): 223–7, 1997. The ASCO experience with evidence-based clinical practice guidelines. Smith TJ, Somerfield MR.

Oncology 11: 1361–1371, 1997. Lumpectomy with and without radiation for early-stage breast cancer and DCIS. Marks LB, Prosnitz LR.

Oncology, Huntingt; 11(11): 1697–703; discussion 1707–8. 1997. Anastrozole: a new selective nonsteroidal aromatase inhibitor. Goss PE, Tye LM.

Pathology Annals 1: 239–251, 1980. Histologic grading of breast cancer. Fisher ER, Redmond C, Fisher B.

Plast Reconstr Surg 56(2): 178–181, August 1975. Reconstruction for aplasia of the breast and pectoral region by microvascular transfer of a free flap from the buttock. Fujino T, Harasina T, Aoyagi F.

Plast Reconstr Surg 93: 96–106, 1994. Recurrence of breast carcinoma following immediate reconstruction: a 13-year review. Noone RB, Frazier TG, Noone GC, Blanchet NP, Murphy JB, Rose D.

Plast Reconstr Surg 95(7): 1207–1212, June 1995. Superior gluteal artery perforator free flap for breast reconstruction. Allen RJ, Tucker C, Jr.

Plast Reconstr Surg 97(2): 364–372, February 1996. Comparison of resource costs between implant-based and TRAM flap breast reconstruction. Kroll SS, Evans GR, Reece GP, Miller MJ, Robb G, Baldwin BJ, Schusterman MA.

Proc Annu Meet Am Assoc Cancer Res 38:(A1123) 1997. Preliminary retrospective cohort analysis, Meeting abstract). Hartmann L, Jenkins R, Schaid D, Yang P Prophylactic mastectomy, PM.

Proc Am Soc Clin Oncol 6: 121(A150), 1987. Can adjuvant locoregional radiotherapy, XRT) reduce systemic recurrence in stage I–II breast cancer patients? Recurrence analysis of the British Columbia Randomized Trial. Ragaz J, Jackson S, Le N, Plenderleith, IH, Spenelli J.

Proc Am Soc Clin Oncol 6: 59(A230), 1987. Conservation treatment of operable breast cancer. Habibollahi F, Fentiman BS, Chaudary MA, Hayward JL, Tong D.

Proc Am Soc Clin Oncol; 9: A81, 1990. DNA flow cytometry measurements are prognostic for time to recurrence in node-negative breast cancer patients: An Eastern Cooperative Group Intergroup Study, EST 7186; SWOG 8696; INT 0076), Meeting Abstract). Dressler LG, Eudey L, Gray R, Tormey DC, McGuire WL, Clark GM, Osborne CK, Gilchrist KW, Mansour EG, Abeloff MD, et al.

Proc Am Soc Clin Oncol 12: 56, (A27), 1993. First line chemotherapy with taxotere, T) in advanced breast cancer, ABC): A phase II study of the EORTC clinical screening group, CSG). Fumoleau P, Chevallier B, Kerbrat P, Dieras V, LeBail N.

Proc Am Soc Clin Oncol 12: 60(A42), 1993. Randomized trial of two doses of taxol in metastatic breast cancer: An interim analysis.Nabholtz JM, Gelmon K, Bontenbal M, Spielmann M, Clavel M.

Proc Am Soc Clin Oncol 12: 64(A59), 1993. Tumor size, ploidy, S-phase and ERB B-2 marker in patients with node-negative, ER positive tumors: Findings from NSABP B-14. Constantino J, Fisher B, Gundz N, Fisher E, Mamounas R.

Proc Am Soc Clin Oncol 12: 69(A79), 1993. Adjuvant therapy for node-negative breast cancer: an update of NSABP findings. Costantino J, Fisher B, Wickerham L, Redmond C, Wolmark R.

Proc Am Soc Clin Oncol 13: 64(A58), 1994. Dose intensification and incresed total dose of adjuvant chemotherapy for breast cancer, BC): Findings from NSABP B-22. Dimitrov N, Anderson S, Fisher, B, Redmond C, Wickerham DL.

Proc Am Soc Clin Oncol 13: 65(A61), 1994. CMF added to tamoxifen as adjuvant therapy in post-menopausal women with node-positive, + VE) estrogen, ER) and/or progesterone receptor, PgR) and VE breast cancer: negative results from a Randomized clinical trial. Pritchard KL, Zec B, Paul N, Paterson AHG, Fine S.

Proc Am Soc Clin Oncol 13: 65*(A64), 1994. Empiric prednisone therapy for pulmonary toxicity after high-dose carmustine*(BCNU). Kalaycioglu M, Kavuru M, Tauson L, Bolwell B.

Proc Am Soc Clin Oncol 13: 69*(A78), 1994. Aredia infusions in breast cancer: a Randomized phse III trial to assess delay in progression of bone metastases. Latreille J, Conte PJ, Mauriac L, Koliren L, Ford JM.

Proc Am Soc Clin Oncol 13: 76*(A106), 1994. Adjuvant tamoxifen in breast cancer: Interim results of a Comprehensive Cancer Center Amsterdam*(CCCA) trial. Vermorken JB, Burgers JMV, Taat CW, van de Slee PHTJ, Hennipman A.

Proc Am Soc Clin Oncol 13: 83*(A134), 1994. Correlation of DNA flow cytometry and hormone receptors with axillary lymph node status in patients with carcinoma of the beast. Friedman NS, Friedman MD.

Proc Am Soc Clin Oncol 13: 107*(A230), 1994. Response to primary chemotherapy (PC) increses rates of brest preservation and correlates with prognosis, Bonadonna G, Valagussa P, Brambilla C, Ferrari L, Luini A, Greco M.

Proc Am Soc Clin Oncol 15: 104 (A80), 1996. Her-2/neu over-expression with clinical taxane sensitivity: a multivariate analysis in patients with metastatic breast cancer(MBC). Seidman AD, Baselga T, Yao T-J, Gilewski T, Rosen PP, Norton L.

Proc Am Soc Clin Oncol 15: (A104), 1996. Lonidamine in modulation of response to doxorubicin in metastatic breast cancer patients. Amadori D, Frassineti GL, Nanni O, deMatteis A, Mustacchi G, Zoli W.

Proc Am Soc Clin Oncol 15: (A108), 1996. Three year follow-up of a prospective study of 219 patients with abnormal mammograms who had stereotaxic localization and core needle biopsy of nonpalpable lesions, Head JF, Kleinbeck SM, Hailey MW, Elliott RL.

Proc Am Soc Clin Oncol 15: 117 (A135), 1996. Phase II study of Gemcitabine in patients with metastatic breast cancer. Blakstein M, Vogel CL, Ambinder R, Cowan J, Pearce P.

Proc Am Soc Clin Oncol 15: 121 (A149), 1996. A large, prospective, randomized trial of high-dose combination alkylating agents (CPB) with authologous cellular support (ABMS) as consolidation for patients with metastatic breast cancer achieving complete remission after intensive doxorubicin-based induction therapy (AFM). Peters WP, Jones RB, Vredenburgh J, Shpall EJ, Hussein A, Elkordy M.

Proc Am Soc Clin Oncol; 15: (A203), 1996. Hormone replacement therapy (HRT) in women with previously treated primary breast cancer (Meeting abstract). Bluming AZ, Wile AG, Schain W, Waisman JR, Dosik GM, Olsen GA, Terperning M, McAndrew P, Van Scoy Mosher M, Decker RW.

Proc Annu Meet Am Soc Clin Oncol 16: 128, 1997. Albain K.

Proc Am Soc Clin Oncol 16: 2, 1997. Phase III trial of doxorubicin (A) vs. Paclitaxel (T) vs. doxorubicin plus Paclitaxel (A + T) as first-line therapy for metastatic breast cancer (MBC): An Intergroup trial (abstract). Sledge GW, Neuberg D, Ingle J, Martino S, Wood W.

Proc Annu Meet Am Soc Clin Oncol 16: 130, 1997. Acute myeloid leukemia (ADL) and myelodysplastic syndrome (ADS) on NSABP-B25: An Update (Abs). DeCillis A, Anderson S, Bryant J, Wickerham DL, Fisher B.

Proc Am Soc Clin Oncol 16: 154, 1997. A randomized phase III study of taxotere (T) vs. doxorubicin (D) in patients (pts) with metastatic brease cancer (MBC) who have failed an alkylating-containing regimen: preliminary results (abstract). Chan S, Friedrichs K, Noel D, Duarte R, Vorobiof D, Pinter T, Yelle L, Alkl M, Murawski M, Riva A.

Proc Am Soc Clin Oncol; 16:(A463), 1997. Hormone replacement therapy (HRT) in women with previously treated primary breast cancer Update III (Meeting abstract). Bluming AZ, Waisman JR, Dosik GM, Olsen GA, McAndrew P, Van Scoy Mosher M, Terpenning M, Decker RW, Rosenbloom BE, Wile AG, Schain W.

Proc Am Soc Clin Oncol; 16:A542, 1997. For the North American Vorozole Study Group, Vorozole versus Megace in postmenopausal patients with metastatic breast carcinoma who had relapsed following tamoxifen (Meeting abstract), Goss P, Wine E, Tannock I, Schwartz IH, Kremer AB.

Proc Am Soc Clin Oncol; 16:A544, 1997. Letrozole, a new potent, selective aromatase inhibitor (AI) superior to aminoglutethimide (AG) in postmenopausal women with advanced breast cancer (ABC) previously treated with anti-estrogens (Meeting abstract). Marty M, Gershanovich M, Campos B, Romieu G, Lurie H, Bonaventura T, Jeffery M, Buzzi F, Ludwig H, Bodrogi I, Reichardt P, O'Higgins N, Chaudri HA, Friederich P, Biachoff MA.

Proc Am Soc Clin Oncol 16:A545, 1997. Significant improved survival with Arimidex (anastrozole) versus megestrol acetate in postmenopausal advanced breast cancer: updated results of two randomized trials (Meeting abstract). Buzdar A, Jonat W, Howell A, Yin H, Lee D.

Proc Am Soc Clin Oncol 17: A3, 1998. Raloxifene reduces the risk of breast cancer and may decrease the risk of endometrial cancer in post-menopausal women. Two-year findings from the multiple outcomes of raloxifene evaluation (MORE) trial. Cummings SR, Norton L, Eckert S, Grady D, Cauley J, Knickerbocker R, Black DM, Nickelsen T, Glusman J, Krueger K, for the MORE Investigators University of California, San Francisco, Memorial Sloan-Kettering Cancer Center, NY, NY, Lilly Research Laboratories, Indianapolis, IN, University of Pittsburgh, Pittsburgh, PA, Lilly Deutschland GmbH, Bad Homburg, Germany

Proc Am Soc Clin Oncol 17: A376, 1998. Efficacy and safety of herceptintm (humanized anti-HER2 antibody) as a single agent in 222 women with HER2 overexpression who relapsed following chemotherapy for metastatic breast cancer. Cobleigh MA, Vogel CL, Tripathy D, Robert NJ, Scholl S, Fehrenbacher L, Paton V, Shak S, Lieberman G, Slamon D.

Proc Am Soc Clin Oncol 17: A377, 1998. Addition of herceptintm (humanized anti-HER2 antibody) to first line chemotherapy for HER2 overexpressing metastatic breast cancer (HER2 + /MBC) markedly increases anticancer activity: a randomized, multinational controlled phase III trial. Slamon D, Leyland-Jones B, Shak S, Paton V, Bajamonde A, Fleming T, Eiermann W, Wolter J, Baselga J, Norton L.

Proc Am Soc Clin Oncol 17: A389. Effect of taxol duration of infusion in advanced breast cancer (ABC): results from NSABP B-26 trial comparing 3- to 24-hr infusion of high-dose taxol. Mamounas E, Brown A, Smith R, Lembersky B, Fisher B, Wickerham DL, Wolmark N, Atkins J, Shibata H, Baez L, DeFusco P, Davila E, Thirlwell M, Bearden J, Tipping S, Scholnik A, NSABP Operations and Biostatistical Center, Pittsburgh, PA.

Proc Am Soc Clin Oncol 17: A390, 1998. Improved disease-free (DFS) and overall survival (OS) from the addition of sequential paclitaxel (T) but not from the escalation of doxorubicin (a) dose level in the adjuvant chemotherapy of patients (pts) with node-positive primary breast cancer (BC). Henderson IC, Berry D, Demetri G, Cirrincione C, Goldstein L, Martino S, Ingle JN, Cooper MR, Canellos G, Borden E, Fleming G, Holland JF, Graziano S, Carpenter J, Muss H, Norton L, For CALGB, ECOG, SWOG, and NCCTG.

Proc Am Soc Clin Oncol 17: A476, 1998. A multicenter phase II trial of Xeloda™ (Capecitabine) in paclitaxel-refractory metastatic breast cancer (MBC). Blum JL, Buzdar AU, LoRusso PM, Kuter I, Vogel C, Burger HU, Brown C, Griffin, T.

Nutr Cancer 12(4): 327–332, 1989. Estradiol binding to plasma proteins after changing to a low-fat diet. Ingram D, Bennett F, Wood A.

Radiology 197(3): 743–7, 1995. Breast tumors: comparative accuracy of MR imaging relative to mammography and US for demonstrating extent. Boetes C, Mus RD, Holland R, Barentsz JO, Strijk SP, Wobbes T, Hendriks JH, Ruys SH.

Radiother Oncol 26: 104–110, 1993. Adjuvant radiation therapy versus surgery alone in operable breast cancer: long-term follow-up of a randomized clinical trial. Rutqvist LE, Pettersson D, Johansson H.

Radiology Clin N Amer 301: 187–210, 1992. Update of the Swedish Two-county program of mammographic scrreening for breast cancer. Tabar L, Fagerberg G, Duffy SW, Day NE, Gad A, Grontoft O.

Science 268: 1749–1753, 1995. A single ataxia talengectasia gene with a product similar to PI is similar a PI-3 kinase. Savitsky K, Bar-Shira A, Gilad S, Rotman G, Ziv Y, Vanagaite L, et al.

Semin Oncol 22: 17–21, 1995. Review of docetaxel (Taxotere), a highly active new agent for the treatment of metastatic breast cancer. Ravdin PM, Valero V.

Semin Oncol 22: 17–20, 1995. The use of mitoxantrone in the treatment of breast cancer. Hainsworth JD.

Semin Oncol 22: 17–28, 1995. Multiple drug resistance: biologic basis and clinical significance in renal-cell carcinoma. Chapman AE, Goldstein LJ.

Semin Oncol 22: 17–21, 1995. Docetaxel (Taxotere): an overview of first-line monotherapy. Trudeau ME.

Semin Oncol 22: 17–21, 1995. Feasibility and pharmacokinetics of paclitaxel, carboplatin, and concurrent radiotherapy for regionally advanced squamous cell carcinoma of the head and neck and for regionally advanced non-small cell lung cancer, Aisner J, Belani CP, Kearns C, Conley B, Hiponia D, Engstrom C, Zuhowski E, Egorin MJ.

Semin Surg Oncol 12(5): 321–327, September 1996. Axillary dissection: when and how radical? Morrow M.

Surg Gynecol Obstet 64: 593–603, 1937. Mammography. Hicken NF.

Surg Gynecol Obstet 129: 705–716, 1969. Location of breast carcinoma and prognosis. Fisher B, Slack NH, Ausman RK, Bross ID.

Surg Gynecol Obstet 140: 528–534, 1975. Ten year follow-up results of patients with carcinoma of the breast in a co-operative clinical trial evaluating surgical adjuvant chemotherapy. Fisher B, Slack N, Katrych D, Wolmark N.

Surg Clin North Am 70: 853–871, 1990. Duct carcinoma in situ Pathology and treatment. Lagios MD.

WHO-Geneva 2: 13–18, 1968. Histological typing of proliferative conditions and tumours of the breast. Scarff RW, Torloni H.

World J Surg 18: 21–31, 1994. Hereditary breast cancer and family cancer syndromes. Lynch HT, Lynch J, Conway T, Watson P, Feunteun J, Lenoir G, Narod S, Fitzgibbons R, Jr.